SECONDHAND SMOKE EXPOSURE TRIGGERED RESPIRATORY CARDIOTHORACIC DISEASES

Secondhand smoke exposure induces harmful health

JIA-PING WU

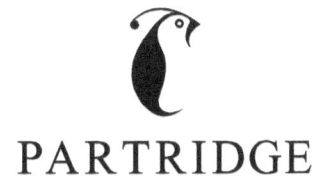

PARTRIDGE

Copyright © 2021 by Jia-Ping Wu.

Library of Congress Control Number:		2020924972
ISBN:	Softcover	978-1-5437-6251-8
	eBook	978-1-5437-6252-5

All rights reserved. No part of this book may be used or reproduced by any means, graphic, electronic, or mechanical, including photocopying, recording, taping or by any information storage retrieval system without the written permission of the author except in the case of brief quotations embodied in critical articles and reviews.

Because of the dynamic nature of the Internet, any web addresses or links contained in this book may have changed since publication and may no longer be valid. The views expressed in this work are solely those of the author and do not necessarily reflect the views of the publisher, and the publisher hereby disclaims any responsibility for them.

Print information available on the last page.

To order additional copies of this book, contact
Toll Free +65 3165 7531 (Singapore)
Toll Free +60 3 3099 4412 (Malaysia)
orders.singapore@partridgepublishing.com

www.partridgepublishing.com/singapore

Contents

Chapter 1: Secondhand Smoke Exposure Accelerates Heart Diseases...1
   Abstract 1
   1.1. Introduction 2
   1.2. Secondhand Smoke (SHS) Exposure 4
   1.3. The Elderly Exposure to SHS 5
   1.4. SHS exposure and Physiological Aging Heart 8
   1.5. SHS Exposure and Pathological Aging Heart 13
   1.6. SHS Exposure and Sarcopenia 19
   1.7. SHS Exposure and Rheumatoid Arthritis (RA) Patients.....20
   1.8. Nicotine and Cardiovascular Disease Cancer 22
   1.9. SHS Exposure and Cardiac Remodeling 26
Conclusion 29
References 31

Chapter 2: Secondhand Smoke Exposure Accelerates Lung Diseases ...53
   Abstract 53
   1.1. Introduction 54
   1.2. Smoking and Secondhand Smoke (SHS) exposure............60
   1.3. SHS Exposure Cause of the Human Chronic
        Obstructive Pulmonary Disease (COPD) 62
   1.4. SHS Exposure Induces Lung Cancer 64
   1.5. Lung Cancer..76
   1.6. The Role of Nicotine through HDAC Induces Lung
        Cancer Growth..81
   1.7. Lung Cancer with Chemotherapy-Resistant Phenotype 90
Conclusion 93
References 95

Chapter 1

Secondhand Smoke Exposure Accelerates Heart Diseases

Jia-Ping Wu
Research Center for Healthcare Industry Innovation
National Taipei University of Nursing and Health Sciences

Chapter 1

Secondhand Smoke Exposure Accelerates Heart Diseases

Abstract

Secondhand smoke exposure and aging cause synergistic effects on the activation of heart-adaptive mechanisms. Active cigarette smoking influences all these pathways. Secondhand smoke exposure always makes for human pathological cardiac hypertrophy. In left-ventricular individual, secondhand smoke exposure may stimuli or first induce a phase of cardiac hypertrophy. Secondhand smoke increases arterial stiffness and coronary cardiac disease events. Secondhand smoke exposure involves the combination of the smoke emitted by the burning end of a tobacco cigarette and the smoke exhaled by the smoker into the environment. Left ventricular pathological hypertrophy caused by secondhand smoke exposure was observed in old-age patients, which leads to left ventricular remodeling and loss of function. Left ventricular pathological hypertrophy leads to ventricular remodeling and increases the risk of a cardiovascular event and mortality.

Keywords: secondhand smoke exposure, aging, heart adaptive, pathological cardiac hypertrophy, smoke, left ventricular pathological hypertrophy

1.1. Introduction

Secondhand smoke exposure has been linked to harmful health outcome which is an important cause of short life span, morbidity, and mortality. However, it is not clear in the pathological condition in old man exposure to secondhand smoke. This report reviews secondhand smoke exposure to old age to determine health mechanisms of the heart. Secondhand smoke exposure increases primary progressive atherosclerosis and arterial stiffness, increases risk of coronary disease events, and causes human diseases, especially in elderly. Aging is a physiology process involving progressive impairment of normal heart functions caused by an increasing vulnerability which reduces the ability of survive. Aging of the very elderly heart is associated with heart failure, an expected or normal aging change. Secondhand smoke exposure involves the combination of the smoke emitted by the burning end of a tobacco cigarette and the smoke exhaled by the smoker into the environment. Secondhand smoke exposure that led to cardiac remodeling has been observed in increasing cardiovascular diseases mortality. nc the elderly exposed to secondhand smoke both at home and outside of the home, exposure at home was higher. Experimental evidence in animal models has indicated attenuation in cardioprotective pathways with aging, yet information regarding myocardial dysfunction in elderly age is limited. Therefore, the numerous molecular and biochemical changes also affect the expression levels of human aging cardiac mitochondrial complex phenotype. Secondhand smoke exposure increases the risk of heart disease, including progressive atherosclerosis, decreased heart rate variability, increased arterial stiffness, and increased risk of coronary disease events. Left ventricular hypertrophy, a condition that has been observed in rabbits exposed to secondhand smoke, leads to ventricular remodeling and increases the risk of cardiovascular events and mortality (1-3). Even for young students, 25.7% were exposed to secondhand smoke at home, 34.2% outside of the home, and 18.3% both at home and outside of the home (4). The old age is a strong independent predictor of death and morbidity in patients with structural heart disease. Therefore, old age is a major risk factor that is associated with poor cardiovascular outcome and that reduces endogenous cardio-protection (5). Both the incidence and the severity of atherosclerosis and cardiovascular disease increase with age. The changes to the heart throughout life are the result of maturational changes beyond sexual maturity, which cause hypertrophy of myocytes and hyperplasia of capillary endothelial cells and interstitial fibroblasts (6, 7). Human cardiac aging generates a complex phenotype (8). Similar data are available regarding age-related changes in the human heart. Secondhand smoke exposure is always associated with age, especially in old age. Age-related changes in an old-aged but otherwise normal heart mimic those changes associated with cardiac diseases, including myocardial infarction, aortic regurgitation, and alterations to cardiac valves and coronary arteries. Age affects cardiovascular function in the same manner as secondhand smoke exposure. Age-related changes in left ventricular morphology and function include decreased myocyte number (9), increased myocyte size (10, 11), increased left ventricular wall thickness, and decreased conduction fiber density, while functional alterations include decreased intrinsic contractility, increased myocardial contraction time, decreased myocardial contraction velocity, and increased myocardial stiffness in left ventricular function. Age affects cardiovascular function in the same manner as secondhand smoke exposure. However, aging also shows relative adaptive responsiveness to eliminate damaged and exhausted cells from birth to senescence (12). Heart failure caused by secondhand smoke exposure was observed in old-age patients, which leads to heart remodeling and loss of function (13, 14). Left ventricular hypertrophy is an initial adaptive response. There are many compensatory mechanisms that respond to increased cardiac workload, sustained left ventricular stimulation being one of them (15). During left ventricular hypertrophy development, there is an imbalance of progressive remodeling at the cellular level (16). Therefore, we aim to further describe the molecular mechanisms involved in secondhand smoke exposure in the elderly to identify the pathological underpinnings of cardiac disease and disorders.

1.2. Secondhand Smoke (SHS) Exposure

Secondhand smoke exposure is associated with elevated risks of coronary heart disease and stroke. The risks associated with high secondhand smoke exposure were very similar to risks from light active smoking, despite the much greater exposure to tobacco smoke in active smoking (17). The mechanisms by which secondhand smoke exposure elevates coronary heart disease risk remain uncertain. However, acute secondhand smoke exposure has been shown to increase platelet activity. Experimental data also suggest that secondhand smoke exposure may cause endothelial damage, increasing endothelial cell turnover and causing a similar degree of endothelial dysfunction to that observed in active smokers. Active cigarette smoking influences all these pathways. Secondhand smoke exposure always makes for human pathological cardiac hypertrophy, but smoking environment in old age health is still unclear. In left-ventricular individual, secondhand smoke exposure may stimuli or first induce a phase of cardiac hypertrophy. Left ventricular hypertrophy has been observed in rabbits exposed to SHS. Left ventricular hypertrophy leads to ventricular remodeling and increases the risk of a cardiovascular event and mortality (18, 19). However, old age is a significant risk factor for cardiovascular diseases (CVDs) (20). Extracellular matrix remodeling is an essential process leading to cardiac fibrosis (21, 22, 23). This is when the extracellular in the left ventricular is now an essential dynamic participant in remodeling (24). Cardiac fibrosis is the consequence of the disruption of the equilibrium between the synthesis and degradation of collagen molecules (25). Myocardial fibrosis results in an excessive accumulation of collagen fibers (26, 27). Secondhand smoke exposure increases arterial stiffness and coronary cardiac disease events (28). Secondhand smoke exposure involves the combination of the smoke emitted by the burning end of a tobacco cigarette and the smoke exhaled by the smoker into the environment (29). Left ventricular pathological hypertrophy caused by secondhand smoke exposure was observed in old-age patients, which leads to left ventricular remodeling and loss of function (30, 31).

Left ventricular hypertrophy is an initial adaptive response. There are many compensatory mechanisms that respond to increased cardiac work-load, sustained left ventricular stimulation being one of them (32). During left ventricular hypertrophy development, there is an imbalance of progressive remodeling at the cellular level, involving cardiomyocyte survival and cell death or cell loss caused by mitochondrial damage (33). Therefore, we describe the molecular mechanisms involved in secondhand smoke exposure to identify the pathological underpinnings of cardiac disease and disorders. In present demonstrate main cardiac hypertrophy signaling pathways, including IGF-II/IGF-IIR/Gαq/calcineurin/NFAT, IL-6/MEK5/ERK5 cascade and MEK1/ERK1/2-GATA4 and JAK1/2-STAT1/3 signaling pathways. Calcineurin/NFAT is originally implicated as pathological hypertrophy signaling pathway (34). On the other hand, calcineurin/NFAT is regulated by MAPKs cascades mediated directly and indirectly. Therefore, calcineurin/NFAT regulating cardiac hypertrophy is associated with MEK1-ERK1/2 and MEK5/ERK5 signaling pathways (35). The subclassified branches IL-6/MEK5/ERK5 pathways have been implicated in eccentric hypertrophy and death regulation in the heart (36). In addition, IL6/MEK5/ERK5 regulates MEK1-ERK1/2 and JAK1/2-STAT1/3 to regulate myocytes growth, apoptosis, and contractile function (37). IL-6 is a pro-inflammatory cytokine, promoting tissue injury and cardiovascular pathologies. IL-6, after binding its gp130 receptor, leads to cardiomyocyte hypertrophy, increased fibrosis, and heart failure (38). In contrast, the JAK/STAT pathway has been elucidated to late essential preconditioning of the heart as well as in cardiac hypertrophy, especially in pathological hypertrophy proves heart function rupture (39).

1.3. The Elderly Exposure to SHS

Aging is an inevitable adaptive human response to exhausted cell, while others regard it as a process that starts at conception and continues until death. Biologists consider aging to be a human physiologic change which has the slowly progressive structural changes and loss in body function with age (40). Cardiac aging is defined as the structural changes and functional declines with the onset of disease or degradation but in the absence of environmental factors, major cardiovascular risks such as smoking, hypertension, diabetes, and hypercholesterolemia (41). Secondhand smoke exposure and aging cause synergistic effects on the activation of heart adaptive mechanism (Figure 1). Genetics and epigenetics also lead to cardiovascular disease, such as heart failure and atherosclerosis. However, aging shows relative adaptive responsiveness to eliminate damaged and exhausted cells from birth to senescence (42). A normal aging heart change, which occurs mainly through from birth to senescence, can produce mimic cardiac diseases, including coronary arteries, myocardial infarction, cardiac valves, aortic regurgitation (43), which is different with heart damage and adaptive response to eliminative damaged and exhausted cells (44). The aging changes of the elderly heart with left ventricular hypertrophy is expected and normal aging change. However, secondhand smoke exposure is associated with pathological secondhand smoke exposure. Therefore, the effect of secondhand smoke exposure in the aged heart is interesting to be revealed. Cardiac aging is a human physiologic change which has the slowly progressive structural changes and functional declines with age, however, which have to in the absence of major cardiovascular risks such as high blood pressure. The physiologic changes of the aging cardiac include left ventricular hypertrophy, increased cardiac fibrosis, and valvular degeneration. However, cardiovascular disease is a major risk factor for aging and cause of death. Aging changes of the elderly heart is associated with physiological left ventricular hypertrophy, which is expected or normal aging changes; however, secondhand smoke exposure is associated with pathological left ventricular hypertrophy (45). Secondhand smoke exposure may lead to cardiovascular diseases, such as heart failure and atherosclerosis. Besides, the effect of secondhand smoke exposure in aged heart is still unclear. Cardiac hypertrophy is a related change in cardiac morphology, including decreased in myocyte number, increased in myocytes size, decreased in matrix connective tissue, increased in left ventricular wall thickness, decreased in conduction fiber density, and decreased in sinus node cell number (46). Secondhand smoke exposure may stimuli or first induce a phase of cardiac hypertrophy, especially in left-ventricular individual. Certain normal aging changes may produce clinical heart disease and may mimic heart disease, such as cardiomyopathy, aortic valve calcium and mitral valve annular calcium. This study found that tobacco use has a significant effect on the acceleration of biological age in smokers. Biological age refers to how old an individual is in terms of his or her health, distinct from chronological age, the number of years an individual has lived. In this study, the researchers ran data on blood biochemistry and cell count results through an algorithm trained to measure age. The administrative data in the study looked at the records of 149,000 individuals; 49,000 of whom were smokers. Their information was compiled as a representative sample of Alberta, Canada, reacting proportionate portions of Alberta's rural, urban, and ethnic populations. Each group in the study also had similar numbers of males and females and a median age of 55. The researchers created age prediction models through supervised "deep neural networks," a kind of artificial intelligence that applies complex math models (47). The study found that smokers showed higher biological aging rates than nonsmokers, independent of other factors like fasting glucose levels or cholesterol. Its models also show that, compared to nonsmokers, female smokers were twice their chronological age. The models predicted that male smokers were one and a half times their chronological age. They also predicted that smokers in the study between the ages of 31 and 40 were biologically older: 44% were between the ages of 41 and 50, and 26% between 51 and 60. The study indicated advanced aging in smokers through 55 years of age. After 55, the researchers note, aging effects curiously vanish. The study suggests different possible causes for diminished effects in older smokers. It could be possible, for example, that tobacco initiates bodily repair mechanisms, which some experts have suggested is the case for smoking and the body's defense against Parkinson's. But it could also be true that the effects of aging, in the long run, are random and psychologically taxing in ways that produce widely divergent individual outcomes, or that many smokers die earlier and aren't accounted for in studies of older individuals (48). Notably, this study is also consistent with recent approaches to aging. We work here reflects the researchers' previous studies on how the advanced technology they use beats chronological age in predicting all-cause mortality and how it can generally track age-related alterations. Other researchers have found the effects of smoking on aging, including one study that used DNA methylation clocks, but this study is the first to use a deep learning-based approach to measure tobacco use and aging.

1.4. SHS exposure and Physiological Aging Heart

Aging is a complex process that is difficult to define. Physiological aging is generally defined to be a decline in body function taking place in the absence of any discernible disease process (49). The process of aging refers to divisions into the young old (65-74 years old), the middle old (75-84 years old), and the oldest old (85+ years old). It is mostly acknowledged that healthy aging of the cardiovascular system is distinct from the increasing incidence and cardiovascular disease with advancing age. Therefore, aging can be divided into two types: physiological and pathological aging. The most well recognized risk factor for many chronic diseases is physiological aging. Interactions between the aging process and the aged-related disease have not been seriously addressed or systematically explained. Aging is an inevitable process of life (50). Cardiac aging is defined as the structural changes and functional declines with the onset of disease or degradation but in the absence of environmental factors, major cardiovascular risks, such as smoking, hypertension, diabetes, and hypercholesterolemia (51). Aging-associated degeneration is a major risk factor for cardiovascular disease. This cardiac physiological aging change include left ventricular hypertrophy, increased cardiac fibrosis, and valvular degeneration. However, the high prevalence of hypertension and ischemic heart disease makes distinction between normal aging changes and the effects of underlying cardiovascular disease processes difficult. Left ventricular aging is a complex process that is still not well understood. Thus, cardiovascular disease is a major risk factor for old age and cause of death. In this study, we focus on aging-dependently physiological cardiovascular outcome. We discuss whether physiological aging of left ventricle (LV) is also associated with cardiovascular disease, hypertrophy, and failure (52). Moreover, we determine aging-related cardiac diseases is associated with numerous molecular and biochemical changes in the heart. Age changes affect cardiac-related protein function and cardiac morphology result in alterations of cell death and survival. LVH is an initial adaptive response to protect heart functions. During LVH development, there are a lot of compensatory mechanisms to increased cardiac workload and stimulation left ventricular sustains (53). Becoming progressively disorganized and degraded with age occurs as a consequence of physiological aging. Aging process can be described as a progressive function decline that leads to the accumulation of errors that damage repair systems and compromise stem cell function. These can cause physical, mental, and reproductive capacity decline through genetic and epigenetic mechanisms, resulting to cell dysfunction. The decline in food intake will make the life span short. This physiological change in aging will take place in older man at risk of developing pathological weight loss when they develop diseases states (54). The phenomena has been described as the physiological anorexia of aging and may be caused by altered hedonic qualities of food, early satiation because of changes in adaptive relaxation, and an excess satiating effect of cholecystokinin. Physiological aging-related diseases, such as sarcopenia and osteopenia, are associated with reduced functional capacity, increased risk of falls, and dependence. Aging or advancing of age is inevitable even in healthy adults. Eventually, they perform certain physical tasks at reduced capacity and in increased incidence of function disability. Physiological aging changes are not caused by disease or environmental influences. Age-associated deterioration is the interaction between genes and environment factors that usually plays the major role in physiological functions rather than genes by itself or environment by itself (Figure 1) (55). Understanding the basic physiological aging processes can decide making sustain quality of life in an aging. Aging is an unavoidable physiological response (56), an inevitable process, random and a passive decline in function, and leads to loss of homeostasis over time (57, 58). This cardiac physiological aging change includes left ventricular hypertrophy, increased cardiac fibrosis, and valvular degeneration. Cardiovascular disease is a major risk factor for aging and cause of death (59). Physiological aging is age-related decline that leads to function decline (60); however, pathological aging is aging-related disease that is aging results in diseases (Figure 2). Diseases that do not occur until or increase in frequency at advanced ages are called age-associated diseases. Indeed, age-associated diseases underlie much of the physiological deterioration of old age. The most well-recognized risk factor for many chronic diseases is physiological aging. Interactions between the aging process and the aged-related disease have not been seriously addressed or systematically explained. Aging is an inevitable process of life (61). Become progressively disorganized and degraded with age occurring as a consequence of physiological aging. Aging process can be described as a progressive function decline that led to the accumulation of errors that damage repair systems and compromise stem cell function (62). These can be caused physical, mental, and reproductive capacity decline through genetic and epigenetic mechanisms result to the cell dysfunction. Because there is a decline in food intake will make the lifespan shorter. This physiologic change in aging will take place older man at risk of developing pathological weight loss, when they develop diseases states.

Physiological aging related diseases such as sarcopenia and osteopenia are associated with reduced functional capacity, increased risk of falls, and loss of independence (63). Although aging is inevitable, with advancing age, even in healthy adults, eventually (64), the perform certain physical task capacity reduced results in increased incidence of function disability (65). Physiological aging changes are not caused by disease or environmental influences. Age-associated deterioration is the interaction between genes and environment factors that usually plays the major role in physiological functions rather than genes by itself or environment by itself (66). Distinctions may be made between "physiological aging" and "pathological aging" (Figure 2). Understanding the basic physiological aging processes can decide making sustain quality of life in an aging. Advanced age is always accompanied by a general decline in organ function even in the absence of overt coexisting disease that do not occur until, or increase in frequency at, advanced ages are called age-associated diseases. Indeed, age-associated disease underlies much of the physiological deterioration of old age. Apoptosis is a recognized mechanism for the elimination of redundant cells in the pathogenesis of cardiac disorders in the elderly. Cardiac aging generates a complex phenotype. Numerous molecular and biochemical changes in the heart are associated with aged-related cardiac disease. These changes affect protein function and cardiac morphology, resulting in alterations in cell death and survival. The biochemical changes also affect the expression levels of mitochondrial membrane free radical changes (67). In aging, apoptosis is upregulated in various cell tissues in a different manner. In myocardial tissue, fundamental processes have been evidenced, independently of the presence of cardiovascular disease, which contribute to maintain the homeostatic state to ensure the normal function. Aging of the heart implies a reduced number of myocytes and of specialized conduction tissue cells, which are not replaced, because of the inability of adult cell to divide. In addition, reduction in Ca++ transport across membranes, lower capillary density, and decreased sensitivity of the cardiovascular system to βadrenergic stimulation characterize this physiological state. Among the molecular mechanisms regulating apoptosis, a role for the pathway PI-3-kinase/AKT-1 has been suggested. PI-3-kinase plays a key role in many cellular processes such as differentiation, mitogenic signaling, cytoskeletal remodeling, vesicular traffic, apoptosis. One of the targets of its specific product PI3 is represented by the protein serine/threonine kinase AKT/PKB (68). PI-3-kinase/AKT1 is reported to deliver a survival signal, giving to the cell the chance to recover from some damage. This pathway seems to regulate the activation of the Bcl-2 family members or/and inactivation of the CED3/ICE family of proteases, as elsewhere reported. The Bcl-2 protein family plays a central role in the regulation of apoptosis. These proteins take part with antiapoptotic (Bcl-2 and Bcl-xl) and pro-apoptotic members (Bax, Bad and Bak), whose reciprocal balance is fundamental in determining cell fate. The final execution phase, when it occurs, results in the activation of a family of proteases, the caspases, which participate in a cascade of events leading to the cleavage of a set of proteins, causing disassembly of the cell. Apoptosis, or programmed cell death, is a recognized mechanism for the elimination of redundant cells in the pathogenesis of human cardiac disorders in the elderly (69). Cardiac TGF-I triggers intracellular signaling cascades that are involved in modulating and facilitating growth and survival and promotes apoptosis (70). In addition, the death-receptor-induced apoptotic pathway, which is initiated by death-agonists and involves the Fas ligand (Fas-FADD-caspase 8-Bid), is reportedly involved in the pathogenesis of cardiac disease (71). Mitochondria may play an important role in apoptosis by releasing cytochrome c, bad, bcl2, and caspase 9 (72, 73). However, caspase 3 apoptosis signaling mediates both mitochondria-dependent and death-receptor-dependent apoptotic pathways (74). In cardiomyocytes, insulin-like growth factor (IGF-I) activates PI3K (phosphatidylinositol-3-kinase)/Akt (PKB, protein kinase B), signaling through IGF-IR and is considered to play a role in preventing myocyte apoptosis (75, 76). The important role of IGF-I and IGF-IR in growth and development and their involvement in the prevention of cell apoptosis have been elucidated. In cardiomyocytes, PI3k activity is required for IGF-I and its receptor (IGF-IR), and PI3K-generated phospholipids regulate AKT activity by direct binding of phosphoinositide to the PH domain. In aging, apoptosis is upregulated in various cell tissues in a different manner.

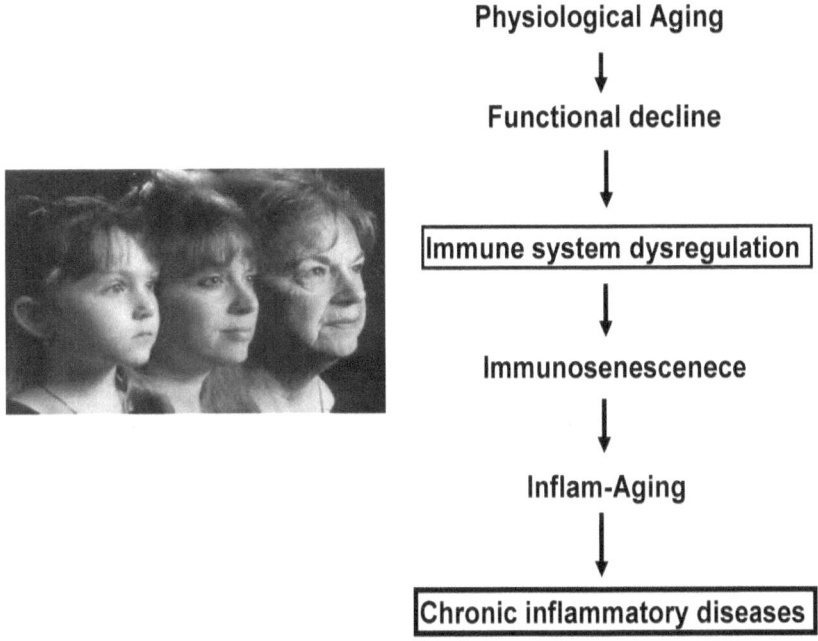

Figure 1. Aging is a physiological process involving progressive impairment of normal functions, caused by an increasing vulnerability to injuries, which reduces the ability of the organism to survive. Obviously, this impairment takes place in a different manner depending on cell type and species. Dietary and environmental factors are the underlying effects of added diseases to analyze that the normal aging process is very difficult.

1.5. SHS Exposure and Pathological Aging Heart

Aging is an unavoidable physiology process leading to random and passive loss of homeostasis in function. Over time involving progressive impairment of normal heart function due to an increasing vulnerability, which reduces the ability of survive. However, it is not clear pathological condition in aging exposure to secondhand smoke exposure. Aging is considered as a major risk factor in cardiovascular disease. Various age-associated changes in the cardiovascular system may lead to pathological outcomes, including cardiomyocyte death, arterial stiffening, myocardial hypertrophy, and desensitization of β-adrenergic, signaling specifically by alterations in structure and function of the heart and vasculature that will ultimately affect cardiovascular performance. Cardiac remodeling during aging includes cardiomyocyte loss, reactive hypertrophy of the remaining cells, and increased interstitial tissues. These changes may result in a decline in the biological and physiological functions of the heart. It has been suggested that the aging-induced cardiac changes render the heart more susceptible to ischemic damage (77). Observational studies have reported that intrinsic cardiac aging is a human physiologic change which has the slowly progressive structural changes and functional declines with age, however, which in the absence of major cardiovascular risks. One of the major difficulties encountered in the study of the effects of age on the cardiovascular system is the differentiation of the aging process itself from the presence of specific disease states. Atherosclerosis, diabetes, and ischemic heart disease are common events in humans, and the severity of these pathological conditions increases with age. Moreover, remodeling of the heart that occurs with advancing age may be in response to left ventricle hypertrophy and increased wall stress and observed with early heart failure and increased fibrosis (78). Therefore, the normal old-age heart changes can mimic cardiac disease. Age-related diseases were also accompanied with an augmentation of fibrotic area and muscle fiber architectural rearrangements in the ventricular myocardium (79). Remodeling of the aging left ventricle typically involves a large net loss of active cardiac myocytes, reactive left ventricle of the remaining cells, and increased accumulation of connective tissue (80). At the same time, the mechanism responsible for the left ventricular fibrosis in the senescent is unclear. These myocardial mechanical properties will result from alternation of collagen. Myocardial collagen is affected by aging process (81). The matrix metaloproteinases (MMP2 and MMP9) are responsible for extracellular collagen degradation and remodeling. The roles of TGF-β1 and MMPs (MMP2 and MMP9) in left ventricular remodeling are intertwined. Both proteins are complex for fibrosis, and both concentrations were elevated. However, the activities of MMPs are regulated by TIMPs (82). Moreover, TGF-β1 is induction through connective tissue growth factor to up-regulate pro-fibrotic proteins (83). Aging is a human inevitable adaptive response to exhausted cells, while others regard it as a process that starts at conception and continues until death. Biologists consider aging to be a human physiologic change which has the slowly progressive structural changes and loss in body function with age (84). Successful aging is the accumulation of the gradual structural changes in people over time but are not caused by disease or disability-free life well through their later years and that eventually leads to death (85). Successful aging is an important part of human societies, referring to a multidimensional process of physical and cognitive capacity, reflecting not only the biological changes that occur (86) but also reflecting the cultural and societal conventions even late in life, existing potential for physical, mental, and social growth and development (87). We can define successful aging consists of low probability of disease or disability over the age of 75 as rated by a physician and have subjective health assessment, good mental health, and high cognitive and physical function capacity (88); active engagement with life, friendship, social contacts, hobbies, community service activities. Life span extension can be established by support system of family, friends, and health care providers (89), together with focus on good nutrition and lifestyle habits and good stress management, can prevent disease and lessen the impact of chronic conditions. A shortened lifespan can occur as the result of genetic alterations; thus, increased DNA repair, reduced oxidative damage, or reduced cell suicide caused by DNA damage can prolong life span. Health aging is the gradual bodily structural change that occurs with time but is are not caused by disease or other gross accident and that eventually leads to death. After the normal transition time aging, an individual is more prone to have problems with the various body functions and develop disease (90). Thus, ageing-related changes may lead to any number of chronic or fatal diseases, such as Alzheimer's, cancer, diabetes, and heart diseases

(Figure 2). Many problems can be caused by aging-related changes. The cardiovascular and digestive systems are particularly affected. Cardiac aging is a human physiological change which has the slowly progressive structural changes and functional declines with age, however, which have to in the absence of major cardiovascular risks, such as high blood pressure (91).

Successful aging is the accumulation of the gradual structural changes in a person over time, but are not due to disease or disability-free life well through their later years, and that eventually lead to death (92). Successful aging is an important part of human societies refers to a multidimensional process of physical and cognitive capacity reflecting the biological changes occurs, but also reflecting cultural and societal conventions, even late in life, potential exists for physical, mental, and social growth and development (93). Successful aging consists of three components: (a) low probability of disease or disability over the age of 75 as rated by a physician, (b) good subjective health assessment, good mental health, and high cognitive and physical function capacity, (c) active engagement with life, friendship, social contacts, hobbies, community service activities. The interstitial collagen matrix is an important component of the myocardium, which surrounds and supports cardiac myocytes and the coronary microcirculation. The interstitial collagen also maintains the myocytes alignment, the myocyte–capillary relationship, and the heart architecture throughout the cardiac cycle. Therefore, the form and distribution of the connective tissue of the heart is such that it may play an important role in the elastic properties and viscous properties of the left ventricle. The major types of collagen present in the interstitium of myocardium are I, III, and V, with type I predominating (94). In non-human primate myocardium, for example, the distribution of collagen types is as follows, 85% type I; 11% type III, and 3% type V. In the myocardium, fibers which surround large bundles of myocytes and individual myocytes appear to be a copolymerization of the I and III collagen molecules (95). Collagen is the only protein in the organism showing definite age changes. A relationship with the general process of aging has, therefore, been assumed. Physicochemical changes in the chemical and thermic contraction have been demonstrated in collagen fibers of different ages. Moreover, biochemical changes in the tissues such as a decrease in the content of extractable collagen show a relationship with increasing age, and the total collagen content in certain tissues has been found to increase with age (96). To understand the changes in the human myocardial tissue in disease, a knowledge of their detailed structure in the normal state is required. However, there have been few studies on the aging of collagen in the human heart. The aim of the present investigation was to determine the types of collagen, to measure the collagen content and the collagen fibril diameters of the left ventricle of the human heart, and to observe any differences between young and aged. Myocardial connective tissue plays an important role in defining and preserving normal myocardial architecture and function (97). Excess deposition of collagen in extracellular matrix can lead to increased myocardial stiffness and subsequently to cardiac hypertrophy and left ventricular (LV) dysfunction. These pathological changes increase the risk of heart failure (HF) and provide an anatomic substrate for life-threatening cardiac arrhythmias (98). Type I and III collagens are the major fibrillar collagens in both normal and diseased myocardium. Both are synthesized as procollagen with a small amino terminal and a larger carboxy terminal pro-peptide (99). Serum markers of fibrosis reflecting collagen synthesis include carboxy-terminal pro-peptide of type I procollagen (PIP) and amino-terminal pro-peptide of type III procollagen (PIIINP), and degradation markers include carboxy-terminal telopeptide of collagen type I (CITP). Elevations in these fibrosis markers have been shown to reflect intramyocardial collagen turnover. The collagen concentration and the intermolecular cross-linking of collagen increase with age (100). Activated MMPs degrade the collagen network and subsequently result in the loss of structural support, distortion of tissue architecture, wall thinning, and infarct expansion. Collagen is the only protein in the organism showing age changes. Collagen in many organs qualitatively and quantitatively changes with age (101). A relationship with the general process of aging has been assumed. An increase in crosslinking of the collagen macromolecules occurs with aging (102). The total collagen content in many tissues has been found to increase with age, a condition referred to as fibrosis. Myocardial collagen is also affected by the normal aging process. There are provide consistent evidence of an increase in myocardial collagen associated with aging. We also observed that there were greater areas of fibrosis in the hearts of the old rats when compared with those of young rats (103). It is well established that the aging process of the heart is characterized by a loss of myocytes. These reductions occur because myocytes are post-mitotic cells and are not replaced as they die. The loss of myocytes could explain the accumulation of collagen in the walls of the ventricles. Another mechanism for collagen accumulation with age could be inhibition of collagen degradation (104, 105, 106). The collagen degradation process in the myocardium by normal aging which a possible explanation is that it is related to cardiac pressure overload.

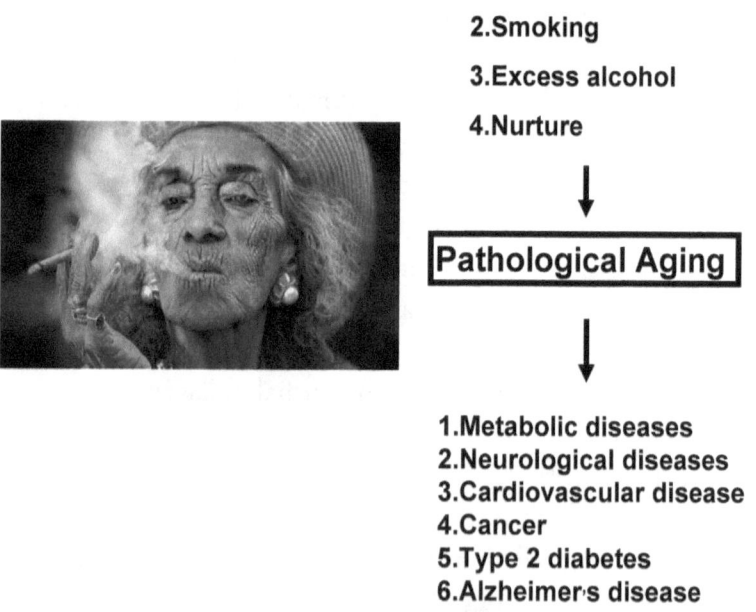

Figure 2. Distinctions may be made between "physiological aging" and "pathological aging." Understanding the basic physiological

aging processes can decide sustainable quality of life in aging. Aging is strongly correlated with a higher incidence of disease disorders, such as cancers, diabetes, Parkinson's disease, Alzheimer's disease, and dementia. Analyzing the normal ageing process free of the underlying effects of added diseases, dietary and environmental factors, is very difficult. The fact that apoptosis is strictly associated with this process in eliminating redundant, damaged, or infected cells is generally accepted. In any case, the complex phenomenon of aging in cells and tissues is associated with number of environment peculiar morphological, histological, genetics, epigenetics, and biochemical changes.

1.6. SHS Exposure and Sarcopenia

Sarcopenia is one of the leading causes of reduced skeletal muscle mass and strength in older adults. Inflammation-aging with aging is known to be a major contributor to sarcopenia. Therefore, sarcopenia has been defined as the loss of skeletal muscle mass and strength in the older age (107). This group proposed that sarcopenia is diagnosed based on a low whole-body or appendicular fat-free mass in combination with poor physical functioning. Sarcopenia is a newly-recognized geriatric syndrome by age-related decline of skeletal muscle plus low muscle strength and/or physical performance through a combined approach of muscle mass and muscle quality (108). This is an importance of sarcopenia in the health care for older people. Sarcopenia starts at approximately 40 years of age, and there is an estimated muscle mass loss of about 3-8% per decade, stretching process speeds up until the age of 70 years; after that age, a 15% loss ensues per decade. Sarcopenia has since been defined as the loss of skeletal muscle mass and strength that occurs with advancing age (109). With aging, sarcopenia has been defined as a syndrome characterized by progressive and generalized decline in skeletal muscle mass and strength, increasing the risk of adverse outcomes such as physical disability, poor quality of life, and death. However, a widely-accepted definition of sarcopenia suitable for use in research and clinical practice is still lacking. Sarcopenia increases the risk of falls and fractures and susceptibility to injuries and can be the cause of functional dependence and disability in the elderly population. However, on average, by 20-40% for both men and women in proximal and distal muscles (110). Thus, defining sarcopenia only in terms of muscle mass is too narrow and may be of limited clinical value that becomes more common in people over the age of 50. After middle age, adults lose 3% of their muscle strength every year, on average, to perform many routine activities. These factors contribute to sarcopenia and to the characteristic skeletal muscle atrophy and weakness. Sarcopenia also shortens life expectancy in those it affects, compared to individuals with normal muscle strength. Aging sarcopenia is caused by an imbalance between signals for muscle cell growth and signals for teardown. Cell growth processes are called anabolism, and cell teardown processes are called catabolism (111). For example, growth hormones are active with protein-destroying enzymes to keep muscle steady through a cycle of growth, stress or injury, destruction, and then healing. However, during aging, your body becomes resistant to the growth signals, tipping the balance toward catabolism and muscle loss.

1.7. SHS Exposure and Rheumatoid Arthritis (RA) Patients

RA status was significantly associated with greater odds of sarcopenia, overfat, and sarcopenic obesity in women but not in men. Among older adult RA characteristics, increasing joint deformity, disability scores, C-reactive protein levels, rheumatoid factor seropositivity, and a lack of current treatment with disease-modifying antirheumatic drugs were significantly associated with abnormal body composition (112). During this time, reduced lean mass, at its extreme termed sarcopenia, and excess body fatness are predictors of poor health outcomes in the general population. Sarcopenic obesity is the combination of muscle loss and fat mass gain; loss of lean mass may lead to weakness, disability, and metabolic abnormalities. Sarcopenic obesity is at its extreme referred to as theorized compound these individual risks (113). Overall prevalence of sarcopenia was 35.4% in women and 75.5% in men, which increased with age. Prevalence of obesity was 60.8% in women and 54.4% in men. Sarcopenic obesity prevalence was 18.1% in women and 42.9% in men. Older women with sarcopenia have an increased all-cause mortality risk independent of obesity (114). Sarcopenic obesity with rheumatoid arthritis and aging, loss of muscle mass as a primary event, and this loss is a major contributor to fat gain, which in turn reinforces the muscle loss. Markedly elevated TNF and IL-1 production in RA, and the various etiologic factors of sarcopenia in aging all lead to loss of muscle. With the increase in fat mass, leptin and TNF secretion are increased, and both lead to insulin resistance, which reduces the normal anabolic effect of insulin on amino acid transport in muscle. In addition, there is some evidence that leptin reduces growth hormone secretion, suppressing another major anabolic stimulus. In addition, higher TNF levels may exert direct catabolic effects on muscle. Obesity in the older adult is associated with poorer performance and strength parameters (115). The purpose of this study is to determine the underlying mechanisms of muscle wasting in sarcopenia obesity patients with rheumatoid arthritis (RA) in the elderly. The abnormalities in body composition and abdominal fat that occur in rheumatoid arthritis (RA) are associated with aging-related presence of skeletal muscle dysfunction (116, 117). Histone deacetylases (HDACs) have been implicated in muscle atrophy and dysfunction caused by denervation, muscular dystrophy, and disuse, and HDACs play key roles of HDACs in muscle atrophy and the potential of HDAC inhibitors for the treatment of sarcopenia in regulating metabolism in skeletal muscle. Several HDAC isoforms are potential targets for intervention in sarcopenia (118). Inhibition of HDAC1 prevents muscle atrophy caused by nutrient deprivation. HDAC3 regulates metabolism in skeletal muscle and may inhibit oxidative metabolism during aging. HDAC4 and HDAC5 have been implicated in muscle atrophy caused by denervation, a process implicated in sarcopenia. HDAC inhibitors are already in use in the clinic, and there is promise in targeting HDACs for the treatment of sarcopenia.

1.8. Nicotine and Cardiovascular Disease Cancer

Nicotine is highly addictive to cardiovascular disease. Nicotine is insufficient as a carcinogen; it functions as a tumor promoter on purpose. It follows that nicotine is only associated with cardiovascular disease in old humans. Nicotine promotes cancer growth (119), angiogenesis, and neovascularization. However, nicotine alone is generally accepted as a tumor promoter but not a tumor initiator in carcinogenesis. Nicotine constitutes approximately 0.6-3.0% of the dry weight of tobacco. Like anything that enters the body, nicotine is also metabolized. Therefore, any activity that increases your metabolic rate can help speed up the clearance of nicotine. Exercise is a good way to increase the rate of metabolism. Exercise improves heart rate and increases the rate of metabolism and burning of heat. For people who have many years of smoking, it is important to start exercising (120). Make sure to drink plenty of water because nicotine is soluble in water, so drinking water helps excrete the substance through the urine. Vitamin A is also helpful in removing nicotine from the body because it also has the effect of speeding up metabolism. Because nicotine tends to destroy vitamin C in the body, it is important to supplement it after quitting smoking.

Nicotine is a nitrogen-containing chemical, an alkaloid, which is made of tobacco plant. Nicotine is also produced synthetically. Nicotine acts as both a sedative and a stimulant (121). Many people smoke, and many people continue their craving for a lifetime. Because nicotine is one of the most addictive substances, one of the important ways to get rid of this bad habit is to get rid of nicotine in your body. Knowing how long it takes and how to speed it up can help you quit smoking sooner. Nicotine enters the body through smoking. In addition to smokers, others inhale nicotine through secondhand smoke. In general, about 1-2 mg of nicotine is taken from each cigarette. After nicotine is inhaled to the lungs, it enters the bloodstream and is distributed throughout the body (122). We all know that nicotine is a toxic substance and is metabolized by the kidneys. Nicotine dissolves in water and excretes through the liver and urine. Most of the intake of nicotine smoke will soon be excreted through the urine. This is also one of the reasons that easily lead to excessive smoking because smokers need to continue to be satisfied. After nicotine enters the bloodstream, it circulates in the body (123). A cigarette nicotine to be completely discharged from the body usually takes six to eight hours. However, nicotine is more present in the heavy smoker. After years of smoking, nicotine deposit are found in fat cells and spreads throughout the body. Once a smoker quits, most of the body's nicotine is metabolized and excreted in forty-eight to seventy-two hours. However, since nicotine adheres to fat cells and other body parts, it takes longer to remove it completely. In addition, cotinine, a by-product of burning nicotine, resides in the body for thirty days. When inhaled, cigarette nicotine will directly go into the lungs. Afterward, oxygenated blood is sent to the brain through the heart. In less than ten seconds, a concentrated dose of nicotine is delivered to the brain's blood vessels and produces a nicotine effect (124). Smoking will lead to lung cancer is an indisputable fact. Tobacco combustion is a very complex chemical reaction process, because of the inability to control these reaction processes, naturally, can't control the production of harmful ingredients. Nicotine is a key factor in smoking addiction. Nicotine is not a carcinogen, but it induces cardiovascular diseases. There is no evidence that nicotine itself provokes cancer. Nicotine binds to nicotinic-acetylcholine receptors (α7nAchR) or EGF receptors, leading to activation of protein kinase B, protein kinase A, and other factors. This leads to downstream effects, such as decreased apoptosis, increased cell proliferation and transformation (125). Although EGFR tyrosine kinase inhibitor leads to a great treatment advance of cardiovascular diseases in old man, only a subgroup with EGFR-activating mutation benefits from it. During the tobacco curing and smoking process, nicotine can be converted to mainly 4-(methylnitrosamino)-1-(3-pyridyl)-1-butanone (NNK) through nitrosylation. In secondhand smoke (SHS) exposure, NNK-induced proliferation appears to involve activation of the α7nAChR, MEK, protein kinase C (PKC), and c-myc. Repeated exposure to nicotine through secondhand smoke (SHS) increases collagen breakdown and transmigration in conjunction with increased tumor growth, vascularity, and resistance to chemotherapy. Nicotine increases cardiovascular diseases and lung cancer cells through activation of the α7nAChR, c-Src and PKCiota. It is suggested that the effects of NNK appear to be mostly dependent upon the α7nAChR. Nicotine binds to nicotinic-acetylcholine receptors (α7nAchR), EGFR, and other receptors, leading to activation of Akt, PI3K, and other factors (126). This leads to downregulation effects of cell growth as well as decreased apoptosis, increased cell proliferation, and transformation. Nicotine also stimulates tumor angiogenesis and cardiovascular disease, which is also mediated through α7nAchR, possibly involving endothelial production of nitric oxide (NO), prostacyclin, and vascular endothelial growth factor. Nicotine might have tumor-promoting or co-carcinogenic activity. Nitric oxide (NO) is synthesized by three key enzymes of nitric oxide synthase (NOS) from the amino acid L-arginine. Inducible nitric oxide synthase (iNOS) is one of three key enzymes generating nitric oxide (NO). Nitric oxide (NO) plays an important role in the physiological and pathophysiological conditions (127). Neuronal NOS (NOS1, nNOS) and endothelial NOS (NOS3, eNOS) are constitutive calcium-dependent forms of the enzyme that regulate neural and vascular function respectively. The third isoform (iNOS, NOS2) is calcium-independent and is inducible. The synthase isoform iNOS is most commonly associated with malignant disease. Nevertheless, the role of iNOS during tumor development is highly complex and incompletely understood. Activity of iNOS has been demonstrated in various cell types, including macrophages, chondrocytes, Kupffer cells, hepatocytes, neutrophils, pulmonary epithelium, colonic epithelium, vasculature, and neoplastic diseases (128). Regulation of NO production via iNOS necessarily occurs during transcription and translation. Once active, iNOS synthesizes large amounts of NO until substrate depletion. Most of non-small cell lung cancer (NSCLC) are unsuitable for chemotherapy remains the cornerstone of treatment for advanced cardiovascular diseases. Platinum-based doublet chemotherapy remains the mainstay for advanced NSCLC. Nicotine binds to nicotinic-acetylcholine receptors (α7nAchR) leading to activation of the Akt. Nicotine can stimulate angiogenesis tumor growth and cardiovascular diseases which is also mediated through α7nAchR, possibly active involving NO and endothelial growth factor (EGFR) (129). Some report indicate nicotine might have tumor-promoting or co-carcinogenic activity. Nicotine is the leading risk factor of lung cancer. Several clinical studies suggest that continuation of smoking during therapy of tobacco-related cancers is associated with lower response rates to chemotherapy and/or radiotherapy, and even with decreased survival. Although nicotine is not a carcinogen, it may influence cancer development and progression or effectiveness of anti-cancer therapy. Several trials have evaluated the influence of nicotine on lung cancer cells. The best known mechanism by which nicotine impacts cancer biology involves suppression of apoptosis induced by certain drugs or radiation, promotion of proliferation, angiogenesis, invasion and migration of cancer cells (130). This effect is mainly mediated by membranous nicotinic acetylcholine receptors whose stimulation leads to sustained activation of such intracellular pathways as PI3K/Akt/mTOR, RAS/RAF/MEK/ERK and JAK/STAT, induction of NF-κB activity, enhanced transcription of mitogenic promoters, inhibition of the mitochondrial death pathway or stimulation of pro-angiogenic factors. These mechanisms underlying nicotine's influence on biology of lung cancer cells and the effectiveness of anti-cancer therapy. Smoking is a major cause of human lung cancer and cardiovascular disease. However, the mechanism by which nicotine induces cardiovascular disease to the cancer remains obscure, although in nicotine carcinogenesis, promotion co-carcinogenesis may have crucial roles. Nicotine exhibits co-carcinogenic and promoting activities in tumor production and malignant transformation (131). Nicotine promoted NSCLC lung cancer in all patients, the role of nicotine underlying mechanisms through α7nAChR nicotine receptor signaling in lung cancer in old man is still unknown. Primary results showed nicotine promoted α7nAChR, NOS2, EGFR and cell cycle-related protein, Cyclin D1/pRb and Cyclin E/E2F increases. Therefore, we suggest nicotine promoted cell cycle actives through receptor α7nAChR or EGFR induced. In the present study, we also want to know nicotine related into cell cytoplasm and nuclear regulation (132). Low concentration level of nicotine increases migration and invasion of lung cancer cells through activation of the α7nAChR, c-Src, and PKC. Nicotine binds to nicotinic-acetylcholine receptors (α7nAchR), EGFR and other receptors, leading to activation of the Akt, PI3K and other factors. On the other hand, nicotine directly regulated NOS2 expression in a α7nAchR dependent manner. Its activation resulted in regression of tumor cell growth and inactivation of cellular apoptosis via DNA damage to α7nAchR and CKЦ α activation in lung cancer cells in the elderly. A time-dependent nicotine treatment induced NOS2 expression and p-Akt increases. Because frequent loss of function of the NOS2 protein by nitrosylation was reported in lung cancer, the nicotine-mediated induction of NOS2 may provide one of its links to α7nAchR. Smoker or nicotine exposure may affect either cardiovascular disease or cancer cells (140). Furthermore, cell membrane receptor proteins, α7nAChR and EGFR, related-nicotine effects. This effects maybe is time-dependent and dose-dependent to regulate NSCLC cell growth. That is our anticipated results and want to resolve. Intricately, we can use these findings to help develop new drugs.

1.9. SHS Exposure and Cardiac Remodeling

Secondhand smoke exposure is the risk of coronary heart disease. In the previous studies, the effects of secondhand smoke exposure on the cardiovascular system include atherosclerosis, increased arterial stiffness, and coronary cardiac disease events (141). Secondhand smoke exposure is the combination of smoke given off by the burned end of a tobacco or cigarette product to exposure to environment and the smoke exhaled by the smoker (142). Most of secondhand smoke exposure is harmful and cause human diseases, especially in children (143, 144). However, it is unclear if low-level chronic cigarette smoke exposure is harmful to older adults. Hypertrophy is an initial adaptive response. There are much compensatory mechanisms to increase cardiac workload and stimulation of left ventricular sustains (145). However, aging is a progressive disease which is the typic natural course who the worsening of the disease until death occurs. Slowly progressive age-related diseases are also chronic diseases; many are also degenerative diseases. However, a static disease exists as a medical condition. Age is the accumulation of changes in a person over time from birth. Aging changes that all people share is universal aging, but someone grow older including disease is probabilistic aging. A mature organism that occurs normally the gradual changes in the structure over time and increase the probability of death. This growing process is unavoidable. This physiologic changes of old cardiac includes left ventricular hypertrophy, increased cardiac fibrosis and valvular degeneration. Cardiovascular disease is a major risk factor for aging cause of death. Aging changes of the elderly heart is associated with physiological left ventricular hypertrophy. However, secondhand smoke exposure is associated with pathological left ventricular hypertrophy (146). Secondhand smoke exposure maybe leads to cardiovascular diseases such as heart failure and atherosclerosis. Secondhand smoke exposure in old heart is still unclear. Heart failure is a related change in cardiac morphology, including decreased in myocyte number, increased in myocytes size, decreased in matrix connective tissue, increased in left ventricular wall thickness, increased in conduction fiber density, and decreased in sinus node cell number. Secondhand smoke exposure may stimuli first induce a phase of cardiac hypertrophy, especially in left ventricles individual. Health aging changes may produce clinical heart disease and may mimic heart disease, such as cardiomyopathy, aortic valve calcium and mitral valve annular calcium. Therefore, we detected the molecular mechanisms behind the aging in secondhand smoke exposure treatment to identify pathological of cardiac disease disorder and elusive. Aging is a physiological process which is from birth to aging the heart undergoes functional changes and which reflect biochemical and ultrastructural modifications, involving progressive impairment of normal functions. Aging of the heart is associated with number of characteristic morphological, histological, and biochemical changes. Because the contribution of these variables to the alterations of the aged myocardium cannot easily be separated from the aging phenomenon alone, the changes of the heart throughout life are therefore the result of multifactorial events in which aging plays an important but indistinguishable role.

Conclusion

The general public have been aware of the harmful effects of tobacco for years now, recognizing its links to cardiovascular problems, cancer, and an array of other serious health problems. The Centers for Disease Control states that cigarette smoking accounts for over 480,000 deaths every year in the United States and seven million deaths worldwide annually, which makes smoking the leading cause of preventable death in the world. Of those 480,000 deaths per year in the United States, the CDC includes more than 41,000 deaths resulting from secondhand smoke exposure. Secondhand smoke can cause or worsen a wide range of damaging health effects in children and adults, including lung cancer, respiratory infections, and asthma. Scientists have concluded secondhand smoke is consent. Children and others exposed to secondhand smoke up the same consequences but did not intend to smoke at all. Cigarette smoking results in deaths annually, 1,300 deaths every day. On average, smokers die ten years earlier than nonsmokers. Unfortunately for individuals who are smoking or exposed to cigarettes, new research indicates that tobacco use contributes to yet another health problem: biological aging. Previously, studies on the effects of tobacco use on aging have been fairly limited in their conclusions, but in recent years, researchers have focused more on the question, applying new scientific tools in their work. One recent study used artificial intelligence to analyze blood and cell counts of smokers and nonsmokers and to measure how much tobacco use aged smokers.

References

1. Ambrose, J. A.; Barua, R. S. *The Pathophysiology of Cigarette Smoking and Cardiovascular Disease: An Update.* J Am Coll Cardiol. 2004;43:1731-7.

2. Antonov, I.B.; Kozlov, K. L., Linkova, N. S.; Paltseva, E. M., Kykanova, E. O. *Aging of the Myocardium and Dilated Cardiomyopathy: Morphological and Molecular Aspects.* Adv Gerontol. 2017;30:282-290.

3. Atteya, G.; Lampert, R. *Sudden Cardiac Death in Genetic Cardiomyopathies.* Card Electrophysiol Clin. 2017;9:581-603.

4. Ayyadevara, S.; Mercanti, F.; Wang, X.; Mackintosh, S. G.; Tackett, A. J.; Prayaga, S. V.; et al. *Age- and Hypertension-Associated Protein Aggregates in Mouse Heart Have Similar Proteomic Profiles.* Hypertension. 2016;67:1006-13.

5. Bernardo, B. C.; Weeks, K. L.; Pretorius, L.; McMullen, J. R. *Molecular Distinction between Physiological and Pathological Cardiac Hypertrophy: Experimental Findings and Therapeutic Strategies.* Pharmacol Ther. 2010;128:191-227.

6. Bernhard, D.; Moser, C.; Backovic, A.; Wick, G. *Cigarette Smoke—An Aging Accelerator?* Exp Gerontol. 2007;42:160-5.

7. Biernacka, A., Frangogiannis, N. G. *Aging and Cardiac Fibrosis.* Aging Dis. 2011;2:158-173.

8. Bisping, E.; Ikeda, S.; Sedej, M.; Wakula, P.; McMullen, J. R.; Tarnavski, O.; et al. *Transcription Factor GATA4 Is Activated but Not Required for Insulin-Like Growth Factor 1 (IGF1)-Induced Cardiac Hypertrophy.* J Biol Chem. 2012;287:9827-34.

9. Bisping, E.; Ikeda, S.; Kong, S. W.; Tarnavski, O.; Bodyak, N.; McMullen, J. R.; et al. *Gata4 Is Required for Maintenance of Postnatal Cardiac Function and Protection from Pressure Overload-Induced Heart Failure.* Proc Natl Acad Sci USA. 2006;103:14471-6.

10. Briguori, C.; Betocchi, S.; Manganelli, F.; Gigante, B.; Losi, M. A.; Ciampi, Q.; et al. *Determinants and Clinical Significance of Natriuretic Peptides and Hypertrophic Cardiomyopathy.* Eur Heart J. 2001;22:1328-36.

11. Brunekreef, B.; Beelen, R.; Hoek, G.; Schouten, L.; Bausch-Goldbohm, S.; Fischer, P.; et al. Effects of Long-Term Exposure to Traffic-Related Air Pollution on Respiratory and Cardiovascular Mortality in the Netherlands: The NLCS-AIR study. Res Rep Health Eff Inst. 2009;139:5-71.

12. Boczonadi, V.; Giunta, M.; Lane, M.; Tulinius, M.; Schara, U.; Horvath, R. *Investigating the Role of the Physiological Isoform Switch of Cytochrome C Oxidase Subunits in Reversible Mitochondrial Disease.* Int J Biochem Cell Biol. 2015;63:32-40.

13. Bonner, M. R.; Nie, J.; Han, D.; Vena, J. E.; Rogerson, P.; Muti, P.; Trevisan, M.; et al. *Secondhand Smoke Exposure in Early Life and the Risk of Breast Cancer among Never Smokers (United States).* Cancer Causes Control. 2005;16:683-9.

14. Bueno, O. F.; Molkentin, J. D. *Involvement of Extracellular Signal-Regulated Kinases 1/2 in Cardiac Hypertrophy and Cell Death.* Circ Res. 2002;91:776-81.

15. Bujak, M.; Kweon, H. J.; Chatila, K.; Li, N.; Taffet, G.; Frangogiannis, N. G. *Aging-Related Defects Are Associated with Adverse Cardiac Remodeling in a Mouse Model of Reperfused Myocardial Infarction.* J Am Coll Cardiol. 2008;51:1384-92.

16. Cai, Y.; Yu, S. S.; Chen, T. T.; Gao, S.; Geng, B.; Yu, Y.; et al. *EGCG Inhibits CTGF Expression via Blocking NF-κB Activation in Cardiac Fibroblast.* Phytomedicine. 2013;20:106-13.

17. Ciampi, Q.; Carpeggiani, C.; Michelassi, C.; Villari, B.; Picano, E. *Left Ventricular Contractile Reserve by Stress Echocardiography as a Predictor of Response to Cardiac Resynchronization Therapy in Heart Failure: A Systematic Review and Meta-Analysis.* BMC Cardiovasc Disord. 2017;17:223.

18. Chantler, P. D.; Lakatta, E. G. *Arterial-Ventricular Coupling with Aging and Disease.* Front Physiol. 2012;3:90.

19. Cieslik, K. A.; Trial, J.; Entman, M. L. *Aicar Treatment Reduces Interstitial Fibrosis in Aging Mice: Suppression of the Inflammatory Fibroblast.* J Mol Cell Cardiol. 2017;111:81-85.

20. Clark, J. D. III; Wilkinson, J. D.; LeBlanc, W. G.; Dietz, N. A.; Arheart, K. L.; Fleming, L. E.; et al. *Inflammatory Markers and Secondhand Tobacco Smoke Exposure among US Workers.* Am J Ind Med. 2008;51:626-32.

21. Deckx, S.; Heggermont, W.; Carai, P.; Rienks, M.; Dresselaers, T.; Himmelreich, U. *Osteoglycin Prevents the Development of Age-Related Diastolic Dysfunction During Pressure Overload by Reducing Cardiac Fibrosis and Inflammation.* Matrix Biol. 2018;66:110-124.

22. Dove, M. S.; Dockery, D. W.; Connolly, G. N. *Smoke-Free Air Laws and Secondhand Smoke Exposure among Nonsmoking Youth.* Pediatrics. 2010;126:80-7.

23. Eisner, M. D.; Wang, Y.; Haight, T. J.; Balmes, J.; Hammond, S. K.; Tager, I. B. *Secondhand Smoke Exposure, Pulmonary Function, and Cardiovascular Mortality.* Ann Epidemiol. 2007;17:364-73.

24. Faught, B. E.; Flouris, A. D.; Cairney, J. *Epidemiological Evidence Associating Secondhand Smoke Exposure with Cardiovascular Disease.* Inflamm Allergy Drug Targets. 2009;8:321-7.

25. Fiedler, B.; Wollert, K. C. *Interference of Antihypertrophic Molecules and Signaling Pathways with the Ca2+-calcineurin-NFAT Cascade in Cardiac Myocytes.* Cardiovasc Res. 2004;63:450-7.

26. Flouris, A. D.; Vardavas, C. I.; Metsios, G. S.; Tsatsakis, A. M.; Koutedakis, Y. *Biological Evidence for the Acute Health Effects of Secondhand Smoke Exposure.* Am J Physiol Lung Cell Mol Physiol. 2010;298:L3-L12.

27. Frey, P.; Waters, D. D. *Tobacco Smoke and Cardiovascular Risk: A Call for Continued Efforts to Reduce Exposure.* Curr Opin Cardiol. 2011;26:424-8.

28. García-Hoz, C.; Sánchez-Fernández, G.; García-Escudero, R.; Fernández-Velasco, M.; Palacios-García, J.; Ruiz-Meana, M.; et al. *Protein Kinase C (PKC)ζ-mediated Gαq Stimulation of ERK5 Protein Pathway in Cardiomyocytes and Cardiac Fibroblasts.* J Biol Chem. 2012;287:7792-802.

29. Geng, J.; Zhang, Y.; Wang, Y.; Cao, L.; Song, J.; Wang, B.; et al. *Catheter Ablation Versus Rate Control in Patients with Atrial Fibrillation and Heart Failure: A Multicenter Study.* Medicine (Baltimore). 2017;96:e9179.

30. Geng, X.; Hwang, J.; Ye, J.; Shih, H.; Coulter, B.; Naudin, C.; et al. *Aging Is Protective against Pressure Overload Cardiomyopathy via Adaptive Extracellular Matrix Remodeling.* Am J Cardiovasc Dis. 2017;7:72-82.

31. Hao, Y.; Tsuruda, T.; Sekita-Hatakeyama, Y.; Kurogi, S.; Kubo, K.; Sakamoto, S.; et al. *Cardiac Hypertrophy Is Exacerbated in Aged Mice Lacking the Osteoprotegerin Gene.* Cardiovasc Res. 2016;110:62-72.

32. Harvey, A.; Montezano, A. C.; Lopes, R. A.; Rios, F.; Touyz, R. M. *Vascular Fibrosis in Aging and Hypertension: Molecular Mechanisms and Clinical Implications.* Can J Cardiol. 2016;32:659-68.

33. Honsho, S.; Nishikawa, S.; Amano, K.; Zen, K.; Adachi, Y.; Kishita, E.; et al. *Pressure-Mediated Hypertrophy and Mechanical Stretch Induces IL-1 Release and Subsequent IGF-1 Generation to Maintain Compensative Hypertrophy by Affecting Akt and JNK Pathways.* Circ Res. 2009;105:1149-58.

34. Hulsmans, M.; Sager, H. B.; Roh, J. D.; Valero-Muñoz, M.; Houstis, N. E.; Iwamoto, Y.; Sun, Y.; et al. *Cardiac Macrophages Promote Diastolic Dysfunction.* J Exp Med. 2018;215:423-440.

35. Janssen, H.; Dunstan, D. W.; Bernhardt, J.; Walker, F. R.; Patterson, A.; Callister, R.; Dunn, A.; Spratt, N. J.; *English, C. Breaking Up Sitting Time after Stroke (BUST-Stroke).* Int J Stroke. 2017;12:425-429.

36. Jefferis, B. J.; Lawlor, D. A.; Ebrahim, S.; Wannamethee, S. G.; Feyerabend, C.; Doig, M.; et al. *Cotinine-Assessed Secondhand Smoke Exposure and Risk of Cardiovascular Disease in Older Adults.* Heart. 2010;96:854-9.

37. Jefferis, B. J.; Lowe, G. D.; Welsh, P.; Rumley, A.; Lawlor, D. A.; Ebrahim, S.; Carson, C.; Doig, M.; Feyerabend, C.; McMeekin, L.; Wannamethee, S. G.; Cook, D. G.; Whincup, P. H. *Secondhand Smoke (SHS) Exposure Is Associated with Circulating Markers of Inflammation and Endothelial Function in Adult Men and Women.* Atherosclerosis. 2010;208:550-6.

38. Jones, S.; Mann, A.; Worley, M. C.; Fulford, L.; Hall, D.; Karani, R.; et al. *The Role of Transient Receptor Potential Vanilloid 2 Channel in Cardiac Aging.* Aging Clin Exp Res. 2017;29:863-873.

39. Kang, P. M.; Yue, P.; Liu, Z.; Tarnavski, O.; Bodyak, N.; Izumo, S. *Alterations in Apoptosis Regulatory Factors During Hypertrophy and Heart Failure.* Am J Physiol Heart Circ Physiol. 2004;287:H72-80.

40. Kaminski, K. A.; Dziemidowicz, M.; Litvinovich, S.; Bonda, T.; Ptaszynska, K.; Kozuch, M.; et al. *Interleukin 6 Is Not Necessary for STAT3 Phosphorylation and Myocardial Hypertrophy Following Short-Term Beta-Adrenergic Stimulation.* Adv Med Sci. 2012;57:94-9.

41. Kehat, I.; Davis, J.; Tiburcy, M.; Accornero, F.; Saba-El-Leil, M. K.; Maillet, M.; et al. *Extracellular Signal-Regulated Kinases 1 and 2 Regulate the Balance between Eccentric and Concentric Cardiac Growth.* Circ Res. 2011;108:176-83.

42. Keller, K. M.; Howlett, S. E. *Sex Differences in the Biology and Pathology of the Aging Heart.* Can J Cardiol. 2016;32:1065-73.

43. Kodama, H.; Fukuda, K.; Pan, J.; Sano, M.; Takahashi, T.; Kato, T.; et al. *Significance of ERK Cascade Compared with JAK/STAT and PI3-K Pathway in gp130-Mediated Cardiac Hypertrophy.* Am J Physiol Heart Circ Physiol. 2000;279:H1635-44.

44. Kimura, T. E.; Jin, J.; Zi, M.; Prehar, S.; Liu, W.; Oceandy, D.; et al. *Targeted Deletion of the Extracellular Signal-Regulated Protein Kinase 5 Attenuates Hypertrophic Response and Promotes Pressure Overload-Induced Apoptosis in the Heart.* Circ Res. 2010;106:961-70.

45. Kunisada, K.; Tone, E.; Fujio, Y.; Matsui, H.; Yamauchi-Takihara, K.; Kishimoto, T. *Activation of gp130 Transduces Hypertrophic Signals via STAT3 in Cardiac Myocytes.* Circulation. 1998;98:346-52.

46. Kyhl, K.; Lønborg, J.; Hartmann, B.; Kissow, H.; Poulsen, S. S.; Ali, H. E.; et al. *Lack of Effect of Prolonged Treatment with Liraglutide on Cardiac Remodeling in Rats after Acute Myocardial Infarction.* Peptides. 2017;93:1-12.

47. Lee, P. N.; Hamling, J. *Environmental Tobacco Smoke Exposure and Risk of Breast Cancer in Nonsmoking Women: A Review with Meta-Analyses.* Inhal Toxicol. 2006;18:1053-70.

48. Li, F.; Wang, X.; Capasso, J. M.; Gerdes, A. M. *Rapid Transition of Cardiac Myocytes from Hyperplasia to Hypertrophy During Postnatal Development.* J Mol Cell Cardiol. 1996;28:1737-46.

49. Liang, Q.; Wiese, R. J.; Bueno, O. F.; Dai, Y. S.; Markham, B. E.; Molkentin, J. D. *The Transcription Factor GATA4 Is Activated by Extracellular Signal-Regulated Kinase 1- and 2-mediated Phosphorylation of Serine 105 in Cardiomyocytes.* Mol Cell Biol. 2001;21:7460-9.

50. Lin, R. J.; Su, Z. Z.; Liang, S. M.; Chen, Y. Y.; Shu, X. R.; Nie, R. Q.; et al. *Role of Circulating Fibrocytes in Cardiac Fibrosis.* Chin Med J (Engl). 2016;129:326-31.

51. Lips, D. J.; Bueno, O. F.; Wilkins, B. J.; Purcell, N. H.; Kaiser, R. A.; Lorenz, J. N.; et al. *MEK1-ERK2 Signaling Pathway Protects Myocardium from Ischemic injury in Vivo.* Circulation. 2004;109:1938-41.

52. Liu, J. J.; Peng, L.; Bradley, C. J.; Zulli, A.; Shen, J.; Buxton, B. F. *Increased Apoptosis in the Heart of Genetic Hypertension, Associated with Increased Fibroblasts.* Cardiovasc Res. 2000;45:729-35.

53. Li, Y.; Asfour, H.; Bursac, N. *Age-Dependent Functional Crosstalk between Cardiac Fibroblasts and Cardiomyocytes in a 3D-Engineered Cardiac Tissue.* Acta Biomater. 2017;55:120-130.

54. Liu, C. Y.; Lai, S.; Kawel-Boehm, N.; Chahal, H.; Ambale-Venkatesh, B.; Lima, J. A. C.; et al. *Healthy Aging of the Left Ventricle in Relationship to Cardiovascular Risk Factors: The Multi-Ethnic Study of Atherosclerosis (MESA).* PLoS One. 2017;12:e0179947.

55. Manabe, I.; Shindo, T.; Nagai, R. *Gene Expression in Fibroblasts and Fibrosis: Involvement in Cardiac Hypertrophy.* Circ Res. 2002;91:1103-13.

56. Manukyan, I.; Galatioto, J.; Mascareno, E.; Bhaduri, S.; Siddiqui, M. A. *Cross-Talk between Calcineurin/NFAT and Jak/STAT Signaling Induces Cardioprotective alphaB-crystallin Gene Expression in Response to Hypertrophic Stimuli.* J Cell Mol Med. 2010;14:1707-16.

57. Marano, C.; Schober, S. E.; Brody, D. J.; Zhang, C. *Secondhand Tobacco Smoke Exposure among Children and Adolescents: United States, 2003-2006.* Pediatrics. 2009;124:1299-305.

58. Martinod, K.; Witsch, T.; Erpenbeck, L.; Savchenko, A.; Hayashi, H.; Cherpokova, D.; et al. *Peptidylarginine Deiminase 4 Promotes Age-Related Organ Fibrosis.* J Exp Med. 2017;214:439-458.

59. McMullen, J. R.; Izumo, S. *Role of the Insulin-Like Growth Factor 1 (IGF1)/phosphoinositide-3-kinase (PI3K) Pathway Mediating Physiological Cardiac Hypertrophy.* Novartis Found Symp. 2006;274:90-111; discussion 111-7, 152-5, 272-6.

60. McMullen, J. R.; Jennings, G. L. Differences between Pathological and Physiological Cardiac Hypertrophy: Novel Therapeutic Strategies to Treat Heart Failure. Clin Exp Pharmacol Physiol. 2007;34:255-62.

61. McMullen, J. R.; Shioi, T.; Zhang, L.; Tarnavski, O.; Sherwood, M. C.; Kang, P. M.; et al. *Phosphoinositide 3-kinase (p110alpha) Plays a Critical Role for the Induction of Physiological, but Not Pathological, Cardiac Hypertrophy.* Proc Natl Acad Sci U S A. 2003;100:12355-60.

62. Meléndez, G. C.; McLarty, J. L.; Levick, S. P.; Du, Y.; Janicki, J. S.; Brower, G. L. *Interleukin 6 Mediates Myocardial Fibrosis, Concentric Hypertrophy, and Diastolic Dysfunction in Rats.* Hypertension. 2010;56:225-31.

63. Mirotsou, M.; Dzau, V. J.; Pratt, R. E.; Weinberg, E. O. *Physiological Genomics of Cardiac Disease: Quantitative Relationships between Gene Expression and Left ventricular Hypertrophy.* Physiol Genomics. 2006;27:86-94.

64. Muhammed, I.; Sankar, S.; Govindaraj, S. *Ameliorative Effect of Epigallocatechin Gallate on Cardiac Hypertrophy and Fibrosis in Aged Rats.* J Cardiovasc Pharmacol. 2018;71:65-75.

65. Murino Rafacho, B. P.; Portugal Dos Santos, P.; Gonçalves, A. F.; Fernandes, A. A. H.; Okoshi, K.; Chiuso-Minicucci, F.; et al. *Rosemary Supplementation (Rosmarinus oficinallis L.) Attenuates Cardiac Remodeling after Myocardial Infarction in Rats.* PLoS One. 2017;12: e0177521.

66. Nadal-Ginard, B.; Kajstura, J.; Leri, A.; Anversa, P. *Myocyte Death, Growth, and Regeneration in Cardiac Hypertrophy and Failure.* Circ Res. 2003;92:139-50.

67. Nicita-Mauro, V.; Lo Balbo, C.; Mento, A.; Nicita-Mauro, C.; Maltese, G.; Basile, G. *Smoking, Aging, and the Centenarians.* Exp Gerontol. 2008;43:95-101.

68. Nguyen, M. N.; Kiriazis, H.; Gao, X. M.; Du, X. J. *Cardiac Fibrosis and Arrhythmogenesis.* Compr Physiol. 2017;7:1009-1049.

69. Nicolai, S.; Rossi, A.; Di Daniele, N.; Melino, G.; Annicchiarico-Petruzzelli, M.; Raschellà, G. *DNA Repair and Aging: The Impact of the p53 Family.* Aging (Albany, NY). 2015;7:1050-65.

70. Oka, T.; Maillet, M.; Watt, A. J.; Schwartz, R. J.; Aronow, B. J.; Duncan, S. A.; et al. *Cardiac-Specific Deletion of Gata4 Reveals Its Requirement for Hypertrophy, Compensation, and Myocyte Viability.* Circ Res. 2006;98:837-45.

71. Ozawa, H.; Miyagawa, S.; Fukushima, S.; Itoh, E.; Harada, A.; Saito, A.; et al. *Sirtuin1 Regulates the Stem Cell Therapeutic Effects on Regenerative Capability for Treating Severe Heart Failure in a Juvenile Animal Model.* Ann Thorac Surg. 2016;102:803-812.

72. Piek, A.; De Boer, R. A.; Silljé, H. H. *The Fibrosis-Cell Death Axis in Heart Failure.* Heart Fail Rev. 2016;21:199-211.

73. Pope, C. A. III; Burnett, R. T.; Krewski, D.; Jerrett, M.; Shi, Y.; Calle, E. E.; et al. *Cardiovascular Mortality and Exposure to Airborne Fine Particulate Matter and Cigarette Smoke: Shape of the Exposure-Response Relationship.* Circulation. 2009;120:941-8.

74. Pugh, K. G.; Wei, J. Y. *Clinical Implications of Physiological Changes in the Aging Heart.* Drugs Aging. 2001;18:263-76.

75. Raghuveer, G.; White, D. A.; Hayman, L. L.; Woo, J. G.; Villafane, J.; Celermajer, D.; et al. *Cardiovascular Consequences of Childhood Secondhand Tobacco Smoke Exposure: Prevailing Evidence, Burden, and Racial and Socioeconomic Disparities: A Scientific Statement from the American Heart Association.* Circulation. 2016;134:e336-e359.

76. Raizada, V.; Thakore, K.; Luo, W.; McGuire, P. G. *Cardiac Chamber-Specific Alterations of ANP and BNP Expression with Advancing Age and with Systemic Hypertension.* Mol Cell Biochem. 2001;216:137-40.

77. Sanna, B.; Bueno, O. F.; Dai, Y. S.; Wilkins, B. J.; Molkentin, J. D. *Direct and Indirect Interactions between Calcineurin-NFAT and MEK1-Extracellular Signal-Regulated Kinase 1/2 Signaling Pathways Regulate Cardiac Gene Expression and Cellular Growth.* Mol Cell Biol. 2005;25:865-78.

78. Sawhney, R.; Sehl, M.; Naeim, A. *Physiologic Aspects of Aging: Impact on Cancer Management and Decision-Making, Part I.* Cancer J. 2005;11:449-60.

79. Seddon, M.; Looi, Y. H.; Shah, A. M. *Oxidative Stress and Redox Signalling in Cardiac Hypertrophy and Heart Failure.* Heart. 2007;93:903-7.

80. Selvendran, S.; Aggarwal, N.; Li, J.; Tse, G.; Vassiliou, V. S. *The Role of Myocardial Fibrosis in Determining the Success Rate of Ablation for the Treatment of Atrial Fibrillation.* Minerva Cardioangiol. 2017;65:420-426.

81. Selthofer-Relatic, K.; Mihalj, M.; Kibel, A.; Stupin, A.; Stupin, M.; Jukic, I.; et al. *Coronary Microcirculatory Dysfunction in Human Cardiomyopathies: A Pathologic and Pathophysiologic Review.* Cardiol Rev. 2017;25:165-178.

82. Shimizu, I.; Minamino, T. *Physiological and Pathological Cardiac Hypertrophy.* J Mol Cell Cardiol. 2016;97:245-62.

83. Stessman, J.; Rottenberg, Y.; Fischer, M.; Hammerman-Rozenberg, A.; Jacobs, J. M. *Handgrip Strength in Old and Very Old Adults: Mood, Cognition, Function, and Mortality.* J Am Geriatr Soc. 2017;65:526-532.

84. Stessman-Lande, I.; Jacobs, J. M.; Gilon, D.; Leibowitz, D. *Physical Activity and Cardiac Function in the Oldest Old.* Rejuvenation Res. 2012;15:32-40.

85. Stranges, S.; Bonner, M. R.; Fucci, F.; Cummings, K. M.; Freudenheim, J. L.; Dorn, J. M.; Muti, P.; et al. *Lifetime Cumulative Exposure to Secondhand Smoke and Risk of Myocardial Infarction in Never Smokers: Results from the Western New York Health Study, 1995-2001.* Arch Intern Med. 2006;166:1961-7.

86. Sun, L.; Ma, K.; Wang, H.; Xiao, F.; Gao, Y.; Zhang, W.; et al. *JAK1-STAT1-STAT3, A Key Pathway Promoting Proliferation and Preventing Premature Differentiation of Myoblasts.* J Cell Biol. 2007;179:129-38.

87. Sun, M.; Chen, M.; Dawood, F.; Zurawska, U.; Li, J. Y.; Parker, T.; et al. *Tumor Necrosis Factor-Alpha Mediates Cardiac*

Remodeling and Ventricular Dysfunction after Pressure Overload State. Circulation. 2007;115:1398-407.

88. Svanegaard, J.; Angelo-Nielsen, K.; Hansen, J. S. *Physiological Hypertrophy of the Heart and Atrial Natriuretic Peptide During Rest and Exercise.* Br Heart J. 1989;62:445-9.

89. Tang, X.; Chen, X. F.; Wang, N. Y.; Wang, X. M.; Liang, S. T.; Zheng, W.; et al. *SIRT2 Acts as a Cardioprotective Deacetylase in Pathological Cardiac Hypertrophy.* Circulation. 2017;136:2051-2067.

90. Toba, H.; Cannon, P. L.; Yabluchanskiy, A.; Iyer, R. P.; D'Armiento, J.; Lindsey, M. L. *Transgenic Overexpression of Macrophage Matrix Metalloproteinase-9 Exacerbates Age-Related Cardiac Hypertrophy, Vessel Rarefaction, Inflammation, and Fibrosis.* Am J Physiol Heart Circ Physiol. 2017;312:H375-H383.

91. Tong, E. K.; England, L.; Glantz, S. A. *Changing Conclusions on Secondhand Smoke in a Sudden Infant Death Syndrome Review Funded by the Tobacco Industry.* Pediatrics. 2005;115: e356-66.

92. Tong, E. K.; Glantz, S. A. *Tobacco Industry Efforts Undermining Evidence Linking Secondhand Smoke with Cardiovascular Disease.* Circulation. 2007;116:1845-54.

93. Trial, J.; Heredia, C. P.; Taffet, G. E.; Entman, M. L.; Cieslik, K. A. *Dissecting the Role of Myeloid and Mesenchymal Fibroblasts in Age-Dependent Cardiac Fibrosis.* Basic Res Cardiol. 2017;112:34.

94. Upadhya, B.; Kitzman, D. W. *Heart Failure with Preserved Ejection Fraction in Older Adults.* Heart Fail Clin. 2017;13:485-502.

95. Van Berlo, J. H.; Elrod, J. W.; Aronow, B. J.; Pu, W. T.; Molkentin, J. D. *Serine 105 Phosphorylation of Transcription Factor GATA4*

Is Necessary for Stress-Induced Cardiac Hypertrophy in Vivo. Proc Natl Acad Sci U S A. 2011;108:12331-6.

96. Venn, A.; Britton, J. *Exposure to Secondhand Smoke and Biomarkers of Cardiovascular Disease Risk in Never-Smoking Adults.* Circulation. 2007;115:990-5.

97. Wang, H.; Da Silva, J.; Alencar, A.; Zapata-Sudo, G.; Lin, M. R.; Sun, X.; et al. *Mast Cell Inhibition Attenuates Cardiac Remodeling and Diastolic Dysfunction in Middle-Aged, Ovariectomized Fischer 344 × Brown Norway Rats.* J Cardiovasc Pharmacol. 2016;68:49-57.

98. Wilkins, B. J.; Dai, Y. S.; Bueno, O. F.; Parsons, S. A.; Xu, J.; Plank, D. M.; et al. *Calcineurin/NFAT Coupling Participates in Pathological, But Not Physiological, Cardiac Hypertrophy.* Circ Res. 2004;94:110-8.

99. Wilkins, B. J.; Molkentin, J. D. *Calcium-Calcineurin Signaling in the Regulation of Cardiac Hypertrophy.* Biochem Biophys Res Commun. 2004;322:1178-91.

100. XM, Ma, Y. T.; Yang, Y. N.; Liu, F.; Chen, B. D.; Han, W.; et al. *Downregulation of Survival Signalling Pathways and Increased Apoptosis in the Transition of Pressure Overload-Induced Cardiac Hypertrophy to Heart Failure.* Clin Exp Pharmacol Physiol. 2009;36:1054-61.

101. Xueyu, L.; Hao, Y.; Shunlin, X.; Rongbin, L.; Yuan, G. *Effects of Low-Intensity Exercise in Older Adults with Chronic Heart Failure During the Transitional Period from Hospital to Home in China: A Randomized Controlled Trial.* Res Gerontol Nurs. 2017;10:121-128.

102. Yang, J.; Feng, X.; Zhou, Q.; Cheng, W.; Shang, C.; Han, P.; et al. *Pathological Ace2-to-Ace Enzyme Switch in the Stressed Heart Is Transcriptionally Controlled by the Endothelial Brg1-FoxM1 Complex.* Proc Natl Acad Sci USA. 2016;113:E5628-35.

103. Yamazaki, T.; Komuro, I.; Shiojima, I.; Yazaki, Y. *The Molecular Mechanism of Cardiac Hypertrophy and Failure.* Ann NY Acad Sci. 1999;874:38-48.

104. Yamauchi-Takihara, K.; Kishimoto, T. *Cytokines and Their Receptors in Cardiovascular Diseases—Role of gp130 Signalling Pathway in Cardiac Myocyte Growth and Maintenance.* Int J Exp Pathol. 2000;81:1-16.

105. Zhang, H.; Wang, J.; Li, L.; Chai, N.; Chen, Y.; Wu, F.; et al. *Spermine and Spermidine Reversed Age-Related Cardiac Deterioration in Rats.* Oncotarget. 2017;8:64793-64808.

106. Dalle, S.; Rossmeislova, L.; Koppo, K. *The Role of Inflammation in Age-Related Sarcopenia.* Front Physiol. 2017;8:1045.

107. Chen, L. K.; Liu, L. K.; Woo, J.; Assantachai, P.; Auyeung, T. W.; Bahyah, K. S.; et al. *Sarcopenia in Asia: Consensus Report of the Asian Working Group for Sarcopenia.* J Am Med Dir Assoc. 2014;15: 95-101.

108. Zembroń-Łacny, A.; Dziubek, W.; Rogowski, Ł.; Skorupka, E.; Dąbrowska, G. *Sarcopenia: Monitoring, Molecular Mechanisms, and Physical Intervention.* Physiol Res. 2014;63:683-91.

109. Wakabayashi, H.; Sakuma, K. *Comprehensive Approach to Sarcopenia Treatment.* Curr Clin Pharmacol. 2014;9:171-80.

110. Doherty, T. J. *Invited Review: Aging and Sarcopenia.* J Appl Physiol (1985). 2003;95:1717-27.

111. Dieli-Conwright, C. M.; Courneya, K. S.; Demark-Wahnefried, W.; Sami, N.; Lee, K.; Buchanan, T. A.; et al. *Effects of Aerobic and Resistance Exercise on Metabolic Syndrome, Sarcopenic Obesity, and Circulating Biomarkers in Overweight or Obese Survivors of Breast Cancer: A Randomized Controlled Trial.* J Clin Oncol. 2018 Jan 22:JCO2017757526.

112. Sanada, K.; Chen, R.; Willcox, B.; Ohara, T.; Wen, A.; Takenaka, C.; et al. *Association of Sarcopenic Obesity Predicted by Anthropometric Measurements and 24-y All-Cause Mortality in Elderly Men: The Kuakini Honolulu Heart Program.* Nutrition. 2018;46:97-102.

113. Emerenziani, G. P.; Gallotta, M. C.; Migliaccio, S.; Greco, E. A.; Marocco, C.; Di Lazzaro, L.; et al. Response to Comment on "Differences in Ventilatory Threshold for Exercise Prescription in Outpatient Diabetic and Sarcopenic Obese Subjects." Int J Endocrinol. 2017;2017:7026597.

114. Chiu, S. C.; Yang, R. S.; Yang, R. J.; Chang, S. F. *Effects of Resistance Training on Body Composition and Functional Capacity among Sarcopenic Obese Residents in Long-Term Care Facilities: A Preliminary Study.* BMC Geriatr. 2018;18:21.

115. Scott, D.; Shore-Lorenti, C.; McMillan, L.; Mesinovic, J.; Clark, R. A.; Hayes, A.; Sanders, K. M.; Duque, G.; Ebeling, P. R. *Associations of Components of Sarcopenic Obesity with Bone Health and Balance in Older Adults.* Arch Gerontol Geriatr. 2017;75:125-131.

116. Delgado-Frías, E.; González-Gay, M. A.; Muñiz-Montes, J. R.; Gómez Rodríguez-Bethencourt, M. A.; González-Díaz, A.; Díaz-González, F.; Ferraz-Amaro, I. *Relationship of Abdominal Adiposity and Body Composition with Endothelial Dysfunction in Patients with Rheumatoid Arthritis.* Clin Exp Rheumatol. 2015;33:516-23.

117. Pecorelli, N.; Capretti, G.; Sandini, M.; Damascelli, A.; Cristel, G.; De Cobelli, F.; Gianotti, L.; Zerbi, A.; Braga, M. *Impact of Sarcopenic Obesity on Failure to Rescue from Major Complications Following Pancreaticoduodenectomy for Cancer: Results from a Multicenter Study.* Ann Surg Oncol. 2018;25:308-317.

118. Lechner, M.; Lirk, P.; Rieder, J. *Inducible Nitric Oxide Synthase (iNOS) in Tumor Biology: The Two Sides of the Same Coin.* Semin Cancer Biol. 2005;15:277-89.

119. Geller, D. A.; Billiar, T. R. *Molecular Biology of Nitric Oxide Synthases.* Cancer Metastasis Rev. 1998;17:7-23.

120. Wink, D. A.; Mitchell, J. B. *Chemical Biology of Nitric Oxide: Insights into Regulatory, Cytotoxic, and Cytoprotective Mechanisms of Nitric Oxide.* Free Radic Biol Med. 1998;25:434-56.

121. Crowell, J. A.; Steele, V. E.; Sigman, C. C.; Fay, J. R. *Is Inducible Nitric Oxide Synthase a Target for Chemoprevention?* Mol Cancer Ther. 2003;2:815-23.

122. Jahani-Asl, A.; Bonni, A. *iNOS: A Potential Therapeutic Target for Malignant Glioma.* Curr Mol Med. 2013;13:1241-9.

123. Liaw, Y. P.; Ting, T. F.; Ho, C. C.; Chiou, Z. Y. *Cell Type Specificity of Lung Cancer Associated with Nitric Oxide.* Sci Total Environ. 2010;408:4931-4.

124. Kleinert, H.; Schwarz, P. M.; Förstermann, U. *Regulation of the Expression of Inducible Nitric Oxide Synthase.* Biol Chem. 2003;384:1343-64.

125. Karthik, B.; Shruthi, D. K.; Singh, J.; Tegginamani, A. S.; Kudva, S. *Do Tobacco Stimulate the Production of Nitric Oxide by Up Regulation of Inducible Nitric Oxide Synthesis in Cancer:*

Immunohistochemical Determination of Inducible Nitric Oxide Synthesis in Oral Squamous Cell Carcinoma—A Comparative Study in Tobacco Habituers and Non-Habituers. J Cancer Res Ther. 2014;10:244-50.

126. Vleeming, W.; Rambali, B.; Opperhuizen, A. *The Role of Nitric Oxide in Cigarette Smoking and Nicotine Addiction.* Nicotine Tob Res. 2002;4:341-8.

127. Chen, Y. C.; Shen, S. C.; Lin, H. Y.; Tsai, S. H.; Lee, T. J. *Nicotine Enhancement of Lipopolysaccharide/Interferon-Gamma-Induced Cytotoxicity with Elevating Nitric Oxide Production.* Toxicol Lett. 2004;153:191-200.

128. Grozio, A.; Paleari, L.; Catassi, A.; Servent, D.; Cilli, M.; Piccardi, F.; Paganuzzi, M.; Cesario, A.; Granone, P.; Mourier, G.; Russo, P. *Natural Agents Targeting the alpha7-nicotinic-receptor in NSCLC: A Promising Prospective in Anti-Cancer Drug Development.* Int J Cancer. 2008;122:1911-5.

129. Nakanishi, C.; Toi, M. *Nuclear Factor-kappaB Inhibitors as Sensitizers to Anticancer Drugs.* Nat Rev Cancer. 2005;5:297-309.

130. Zhang, T.; Lu, H.; Shang, X.; Tian, Y.; Zheng, C.; Wang, S.; Cheng, H.; Zhou, R. *Nicotine Prevents the Apoptosis Induced by Menadione in Human Lung Cancer Cells.* Biochem Biophys Res Commun. 2006;342:928-34.

131. Ho, Y. S.; Chen, C. H.; Wang, Y. J.; Pestell, R. G.; Albanese, C.; Chen, R. J.; Chang, M. C.; Jeng, J. H.; Lin, S. Y.; Liang, Y. C.; Tseng, H.; Lee, W. S.; Lin, J. K.; Chu, J. S.; Chen, L. C.; Lee, C. H.; Tso, W. L.; Lai, Y. C.; Wu, C. H. *Tobacco-Specific Carcinogen 4-(methylnitrosamino)-1-(3-pyridyl)-1-butanone (NNK) Induces Cell Proliferation in Normal Human Bronchial Epithelial Cells*

through NFkappaB Activation and Cyclin D1 Up-Regulation. Toxicol Appl Pharmacol. 2005;205:133-48.

132. Tsurutani, J.; Castillo, S. S.; Brognard, J.; Granville, C. A.; Zhang, C.; Gills, J. J.; Sayyah, J.; Dennis, P. A. *Tobacco Components Stimulate Akt-Dependent Proliferation and NFkappaB-Dependent Survival in Lung Cancer Cells.* Carcinogenesis. 2005;26:1182-95.

133. Ramasamy, K.; Dwyer-Nield, L. D.; Serkova, N. J.; Hasebroock, K. M.; Tyagi, A.; Raina, K.; Singh, R. P.; Malkinson, A. M.; Agarwal, R. *Silibinin Prevents Lung Tumorigenesis in Wild-Type but Not in iNOS-/-Mice: Potential of Real-Time Micro-CT in Lung Cancer Chemoprevention Studies.* Clin Cancer Res. 2011;17:753-61

134. Chang, W. C.; Lee, Y. C.; Liu, C. L.; Hsu, J. D.; Wang, H. C.; Chen, C. C.; Wang, C. J. *Increased Expression of iNOS and c-fos via Regulation of Protein Tyrosine Phosphorylation and MEK1/ERK2 Proteins in Terminal Bronchiole Lesions in the Lungs of Rats Exposed to Cigarette Smoke.* Arch Toxicol. 2001;75:28-35.

135. Simon, P. S.; Sharman, S. K.; Lu, C.; Yang, D.; Paschall, A. V.; Tulachan, S. S.; Liu, K. *The NF-κB p65 and p50 Homodimer Cooperate with IRF8 to Activate iNOS Transcription.* BMC Cancer. 2015;15:770.

136. Sahu, B. D.; Kalvala, A. K.; Koneru, M.; Mahesh Kumar, J.; Kuncha, M.; Rachamalla, S. S.; Sistla, R. *Ameliorative Effect of Fisetin on Cisplatin-Induced Nephrotoxicity in Rats via Modulation of NF-κB Activation and Antioxidant Defence.* PLoS One. 2014;9:e105070.

137. Shaked, H.; Hofseth, L. J.; Chumanevich, A.; Chumanevich, A. A.; Wang, J.; Wang, Y.; Taniguchi, K.; Guma, M.; Shenouda, S.; Clevers, H.; Harris, C. C.; Karin, M. *Chronic Epithelial NF-κB Activation Accelerates APC Loss and Intestinal Tumor*

Initiation through iNOS Up-Regulation. Proc Natl Acad Sci USA. 2012;109:14007-12.

138. Du, Q.; Zhang, X.; Cardinal, J.; Cao, Z.; Guo, Z.; Shao, L.; Geller, D. A. *Wnt/beta-catenin Signaling Regulates Cytokine-Induced Human Inducible Nitric Oxide Synthase Expression by Inhibiting Nuclear factor-kappaB Activation in Cancer Cells.* Cancer Res. 2009;69:3764-71.

139. Dasgupta, P.; Kinkade, R.; Joshi, B.; Decook, C.; Haura, E.; Chellappan, S. *Nicotine Inhibits Apoptosis Induced by Chemotherapeutic Drugs by Up-Regulating XIAP and Survivin.* Proc Natl Acad Sci USA. 2006;103:6332-7.

140. Bard, R. L.; Dvonch, J. T.; Kaciroti, N.; Lustig, S. A.; Brook, R. D. *Is Acute High-Dose Secondhand Smoke Exposure Always Harmful to Microvascular Function in Healthy Adults?* Prev Cardiol. 2010;13:175-9.

141. Dai, D. F.; Chen, T. Johnson, S. C.; Szeto, H.; Rabinovitch, P. S. Cardiac Aging: From Molecular Mechanisms to Significance in Human Health and Disease. Antioxid Redox Signal. 2012;16:1492-526.

142. Faught, B. E.; Flouris, A. D.; Cairney, J. *Epidemiological Evidence Associating Secondhand Smoke Exposure with Cardiovascular Disease.* Inflamm Allergy Drug Targets. 2009;8:321-7.

143. Flouris, A. D.; Vardavas, C. I.; Metsios, G. S.; Tsatsakis, A. M.; Koutedakis, Y. *Biological Evidence for the Acute Health Effects of Secondhand Smoke Exposure.* Am J Physiol Lung Cell Mol Physiol. 2010;298:L3-L12.

144. Michaud, M.; Balardy, L.; Moulis, G.; Gaudin, C.; Peyrot, C.; Vellas, B.; Cesari, M.; Nourhashemi, F. *Proinflammatory*

Cytokines, Aging, and Age-Related Diseases. J Am Med Dir Assoc. 2013;13:S1525-8610.

145. Wu, J. P.; Che, T. T. *Secondhand Smoke Exposure in Aging-related Cardiac Disease.* Aging Dis. 2013:4,127-33.

146. Zhu, J.; Rebecchi, M. J.; Wang, Q.; Glass, P. S.; Brink, P. R.; Liu, L. *Chronic Tempol Treatment Restores Pharmacological Preconditioning in the Senescent Rat Heart.* Am J Physiol Heart Circ Physiol. 2013;304:H649-59.

Chapter 2

Secondhand Smoke Exposure Accelerates Lung Diseases

Jia-Ping Wu
Research Center for Healthcare Industry Innovation
National Taipei University of Nursing and Health Sciences

Chapter 2

Secondhand Smoke Exposure Accelerates Lung Diseases

Abstract

Secondhand smoke (SHS) exposure has been linked to a harmful health outcome. There is an important evidence on cause of morbidity and mortality. Secondhand smoke exposure presents a challenging lung health hazard. SHS exposure, toxic air contamination, causes lung cancer and cardiovascular diseases. SHS is a major cause of human lung cancer, however, by which induces cancer remains obscure; although secondhand smoke exposure extract carcinogenesis, promotion co-carcinogenesis may have crucial roles. Secondhand smoke exposure exhibits co-carcinogenic and promoting activities in tumor production and malignant transformation. Secondhand smoke exposure promoted NSCLC lung cancer in all patients, the role of secondhand smoke exposure underlying mechanisms through α7nAChR. Secondhand smoke exposure receptor signaling in lung cancer is still unknown. To determine SHS exposure induces NSCLC cancer cell lines proliferation, cell growth, and migration using immunoblot and immunofluorescent analysis. Furthermore, we detected cell receptor proteins, α7nAChR and EGFR, related-nicotine effects in the cytosol and nuclear using immunoblot and immunofluorescent analysis. Protein expression levels of α7nAChR, NOS2, EGFR, and cell cycle-related proteins were examined. Primary results showed SHS exposure promoted α7nAChR, NOS2, EGFR, and cell cycle-related proteins, Cyclin D1/Rb and Cyclin E/E2F, are increased. Therefore, we suggest secondhand smoke exposure promoted cell cycle actives through receptor α7nAChR or EGFR induced. In the present study, we also want to know SHS exposure related to cell cytoplasm and nuclear regulation.

Keywords: secondhand smoke exposure, lung cancer, cardiovascular diseases, cytosol, nuclear, cell proliferation, cell growth

1.1. Introduction

Secondhand smoke exposure increases the migration of lung cancer cells through activation of the α7nAChR. Secondhand smoke exposure binds to nicotinic-acetylcholine receptors (α7nAchR), EGFR, and other receptors, leading to activation of the cell cycle and other factors (1). Secondhand smoke exposure directly regulated cell cycle expression in α7nAchR dependent manner. Its activation resulted in regression of tumor cell growth and inactivation of cellular apoptosis via cell cycle inhibition to α7nAchR and EGFR activation in H157 lung cancer cells (2). A time-dependent cigarette smoke extract treatment-induced cell cycle expression and cell cycle increases. Because of lung cancer, the secondhand smoke exposure-mediated induction of cell cycle may provide one of its links to α7nAchR (3). NSCLC cells included adenocarcinoma and squamous lung cancer cells. They are different functions between adenocarcinoma and squamous. Secondhand smoke exposure may affect either adenocarcinoma or squamous. In this study, we determine cigarette smoke extract not only induced squamous cancer cells proliferation and growth but also induced by adenocarcinoma cancer cells. This effect maybe is on time- and dose-dependent regulated NSCLC cell growth. That is our anticipated results and what we want to resolve. Intricately, we can use these findings to help new drug development. Sometimes malignant cancer develops in one part of the body and then spreads to other parts of the body, a process known as metastasis (4). There are currently over two hundred different types of cancer, each of which has its own diagnostic and therapeutic approach. Cancer is a genetic disease, damages DNA caused by environmental exposures, such as chemicals or tobacco smoke. More than 1.2 million people die of lung cancer each year. Lung cancer is also the first frequently diagnosed cancer in Taiwan, and it accounts for 20% of cancer deaths (5). The major patients of lung cancer are non-small cell lung cancer (NSCLC), which comprises approximately 80% of all new lung cancer patients. Non-small cell lung cancer is the most common type of lung cancer. About 85% of lung cancers are non-small cell lung cancers. Squamous cell carcinoma, adenocarcinoma, and large cell carcinoma are all subtypes of non-small cell lung cancer (6). Small cell lung cancer is also called oat cell cancer. About 10-15% of lung cancers are small cell lung cancer (7). This type of lung cancer tends to spread quickly. Lung carcinoid tumor is less than 5% of lung cancers. They are also sometimes called lung neuroendocrine tumors. Most of these tumors grow slowly and really spread (8-9). Despite a large number of clinical trials aimed at improving patient survival, lung cancer remains a leading cause of cancer-related mortality worldwide in both men and women. Notably, lung adenocarcinoma, the predominant histological subtype of NSCLC, accounts for 20-30% of primary lung cancer cases among subjects under 45 years of age, regardless of smoking history (10).

Chemotherapy drugs and target drugs may be recommended. Chemotherapy drugs and similar types of drugs interfere with the way cells work and can kill cells in various phases of the cell cycle. These drugs may be combined to attack cancer cells in different ways (11). Most large phase 3 trials have shown a median survival time of eight to ten months, a one-year survival rate of 30-35% and the five-year survival rate of the late stage of lung cancer patients is 1%. In addition, 30–50% of the patients who present at an earlier stage and are treated initially with surgery or thoracic radiotherapy will die of metastatic recurrence, underscoring the need for more effective systemic therapy. Most cases of NSCLC are unsuitable for surgery, and chemotherapy remains the cornerstone of treatment for advanced disease. Platinum-based doublet chemotherapy remains the mainstay for advanced NSCLC, but toxicities, including leukopenia, nephrotoxicity, or neurotoxicity, hinder its application (12). Although EGFR tyrosine kinase inhibitor leads to a great treatment advance of NSCLC, only a subgroup with EGFR activating mutation benefits from it. Hence, the development of new anti-lung cancer drugs or treatments has become an important and urgent issue. Chemotherapy drugs target cells at different phases of the process of forming the cell cycle (13). Chemotherapy is a kind of drug that kill cancer cells to treat tumors. The main function of these drugs is to inhibit the different parts of the tumor cell cycle. Depending on the effect of the drug on cell proliferation kinetics, drugs that differentiate cell cycle-specific and cell cycle non-specific tumors. Target drugs as a form of molecular medicine targeted therapy blocks the growth of cancer cells by interfering with specific targeted molecules needed for carcinogenesis and tumor growth (14), rather than by simply interfering with all rapidly dividing cells. Antibody-drug conjugates combined biologic and cytotoxic mechanisms into one targeted therapy (15). A drug therapy that blocks the growth of cancer cells by interfering with the specific molecules required for canceration or tumor proliferation. Targeted therapy can reverse the malignant phenotype of tumor cells (16). The limitation of the clinical application of a drug shall be its low side effect and specificity. Thus, we will test their specificities and toxicity with lung cells and other cancer cells of different origins. The prognosis of patients with advanced NSCLC is very poor. Not all cancer patients are eligible for targeted therapy. Targeted therapy may be limited to patients whose tumor site has the proper target for a targeted therapeutic drug to play a role (17). Sometimes a patient is eligible for a targeted therapy only if the patient meets certain conditions (for example, cancer does not respond to other therapies, cancer has spread, or can't be surgically removed). Cancer development is not restricted to the genetic changes but may also involve epigenetic changes. SHS exposure constitutes approximately 0.6-3.0% of the dry weight of tobacco. Like anything that enters the body, nicotine is also metabolized. Therefore, any activity that increases your metabolic rate can help speed up the clearance of nicotine (18). Exercise is a good way to increase the rate of metabolism. Exercise improves heart rate and increases the rate of metabolism and burning of heat. For people who have many years of smoking, it is important to start exercising. Make sure to drink plenty of water because nicotine is soluble in water, so drinking water helps excrete the substance through the urine (19). Vitamin A is also helpful in removing nicotine from the body because it also has the effect of speeding up the metabolism. Because nicotine tends to destroy vitamin C in the body, it is important to supplement it after quitting smoking (20). Secondhand smoke exposure is highly addictive. Secondhand smoke exposure is insufficient as a carcinogen, it functions as a tumor promoter on purpose. It follows that nicotine is associated with cancer in humans. Secondhand smoke exposure also promotes cancer growth, angiogenesis and neovascularization. Thereby, secondhand smoke exposure impeding apoptosis, promoting tumor growth and activating growth factors (21). Secondhand smoke exposure binds to nicotinic-acetylcholine receptors (nAChR) or EGF receptors, leading to activation of protein kinase B, protein kinase A, and other factors. This leads to downstream effects, such as decreased apoptosis, increased cell proliferation, and transformation. Secondhand smoke exposure also stimulates angiogenesis and tumor growth which is also mediated through nicotinic-acetylcholine receptors (nAChR), possibly involving endothelial production of nitric oxide (NO), prostacyclin, and vascular endothelial growth factor (22). HDAC2 and nicotine leading to activation of decreased apoptosis and increased cell proliferation. Various NSCLC cells, HDAC2, Valporic acid, and cisplatin in H157 cancer cell migration distributed of HDAC2 and PARP in the cytoplasm and nuclear in H157 and H520 cell lines. Cell cycle frequency, implicating that might be required for cigarette carcinogenic content-mediated advanced development or treatment failure in total lung cancer cases, regardless of tissue types. Intriguingly, this association seen in smoker and non-smoker groups was demonstrated in only squamous cell carcinoma (SC), but not in adenocarcinoma (AD), confirming the specific interplay between cell cycle and carcinogenic content of cigarette (23). It is that the contribution of the increased cell cycle to a poor survival rate is limited in those smokers with SC lung cancer. On the other hand, those associations seen in relapse and relapse-free patients were observed in all lung cancer cases, despite tissue types, suggesting the critical role of cell cycle in treatment failure/resistance or metastasis of lung cancer. Treatment with significantly increased the cytotoxicity of cisplatin in both A549 (AD) and H520 (SC) cells. Hence, the aberrant interplay of the cell cycle with SHS exposure may be required for its oncogenic activity in SC lung cancer and cell cycle may be required for treatment failure/resistance or metastasis and, therefore, contributes to relapse (24). It is important to disclose such a common protein exerting pleiotropic effects on lung cancer because we may be able to identify individuals with poor outcome in lung cancer patients. In addition, appropriate treatment and prevention can be taken far earlier after/before lung cancer develops. Therefore, we have four major goals to accomplish in this project. This is the very first study linking SHS exposure to cell cycle aberrations in lung cancer. Notably, nicotine constitutes approximately 0.6–3.0% of the dry weight of tobacco (25). The accomplishment of this project will not only provide a better understanding of lung cancer development but also provide useful information for the clinicians to decide the appropriate drugs/treatments for each individual lung cancer patient (26). Our findings suggested that aberrations of the cell cycle may play some critical roles in NSCLC. Thus, with the accomplishment of this project, we may develop a more effective treatment strategy for lung cancer using clinically available cell cycle. SHS exposure is highly addictive to NSCLC lung cancer (Figure 1). Secondhand smoke exposure is insufficient as carcinogenesis, it functions as a tumor promoter on purpose. It follows that nicotine is associated with cancer in humans. Secondhand smoke exposure also promotes cancer growth, angiogenesis, and neovascularization. Secondhand smoke exposure cause of human lung cancer remains obscure, although secondhand smoke exposure induces carcinogenesis, promotion co-carcinogenesis may have crucial roles (27). Secondhand smoke exposure may affect either adenocarcinoma or squamous. SHS exposure is a major cause of human lung cancer (Figure 1). Secondhand smoke exposure is the leading risk factor for lung cancer. Several clinical studies suggest that continuation of secondhand smoke during therapy of tobacco-related cancers is associated with lower response rates to chemotherapy and/or radiotherapy, and even with decreased survival (28). Although nicotine is not a carcinogen, it may influence cancer development and progression or effectiveness of anti-cancer therapy (29). Secondhand smoke lead to DNA damage. Secondhand smoke exposure contains more than six thousand components. Secondhand smoke exposure is the leading risk factor for lung cancer (Figure 1). Secondhand smoke exposure or air pollution appears to be the primary underlying cause of cancer. Chemotherapy drugs and target drugs maybe recommended (30). Chemotherapy drugs, these types of drugs interfere with the way cells work and can kill cells in various phases of the cell cycle. These drugs may be combined to attack cancer cells in different ways. Most cases of NSCLC are unsuitable for surgery, and chemotherapy remains the cornerstone of treatment for advanced disease (31). A drug therapy that blocks the growth of cancer cells by interfering with the specific molecules required for canceration or tumor proliferation.

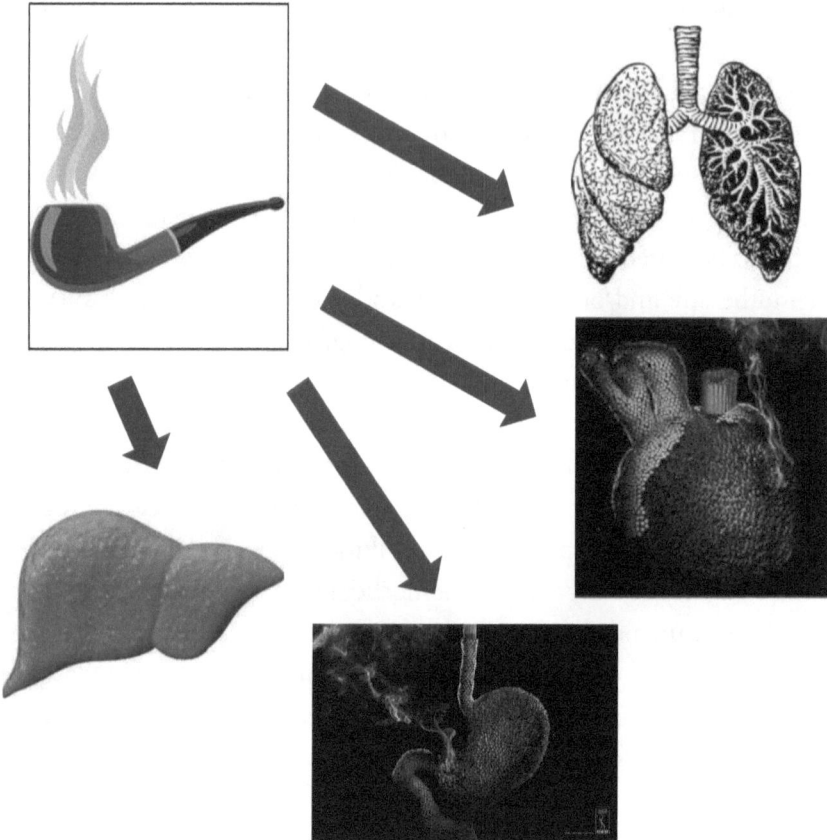

Figure 1. Secondhand smoke contains hundreds of chemicals known to be toxic or carcinogenic. It has been used for treatment of numerous human cancers, including bladder, head and neck, lung, ovarian, and testicular cancers. The standard of care for localized non-small-cell lung cancer (NSCLC) is surgery followed by, in case of stage II and III disease, adjuvant cisplatin-based chemotherapy.

1.2. Smoking and Secondhand Smoke (SHS) exposure

The association seen in smoker and non-smoker groups was demonstrated in only squamous cell lung cancer (SC), but not in adenocarcinoma (AD), confirming the specific interplay between

HDAC2 and carcinogenic content of cigarette. It is noted that nicotine constitutes approximately 0.6–3.0% of the dry weight of tobacco (30). We, therefore, examine its potential impacts on HDAC2 expression or functions in squamous lung cancer cells (H157 and H520). The viability rate of exposure nicotine in H157 cell line with survival is no significant correlation (Figure 1). It is demonstrated that HDAC2 expression was also correlated with TNM stage and negatively correlated with differentiation of NSCLC and apoptotic index (31). The survival outcome of NSCLC cell line with low expression of HDAC2 was better than that of those with high expression. The expression of HDAC2 was found to be associated with most cell types of NSCLC, and nicotine exposure is significantly higher in NSCLC than in normal lung cells. Those associations seen in nicotine and cisplatin treatment were observed in all NSCLC cases, despite of squamous lung cancer cells types, suggesting the critical role of HDAC2 in treatment failure/resistance or metastasis of lung cancer. In addition, increased HDAC2 in nuclear and cytosol may play roles in treatment failure/resistance or metastasis of lung cancer. Various NSCLC cells have an obviously increased HDAC2 expression. The well-tolerated antiepileptic drug, valproic acid (VPA), is a class I selective HDAC inhibitor and selectively induces proteasomal degradation of HDAC2. This activity can be distinguished from its therapeutically exploited antiepileptic activity. Since VPA has been used clinically for over two decades, the pharmacology and side effects of this drug have been studied in detail (32). As expected for HDAC inhibitory compounds, VPA induces differentiation of carcinoma cells, transformed hematopoietic progenitor cells and leukemic blasts from acute myeloid leukemia patients. Moreover, tumor growth and metastasis formation are significantly reduced in animal experiments. Interestingly, VPA was also reported to have beneficial effects for patients suffering from neuroblastomas and glioblastomas even before its HDAC inhibitory properties were established.

1.3. SHS Exposure Cause of the Human Chronic Obstructive Pulmonary Disease (COPD)

Secondhand smoke exposure causes human chronic obstructive pulmonary disease (COPD). COPD, known as lung obstruction, is a common respiratory disease characterized by persistent expiratory flow. COPD is the third leading cause of mortality worldwide. It is defined by persistent airflow disordered that is progressive and associated with increased chronic airway and lung inflammatory responses to noxious particles or gases (33). The primary cause of COPD is tobacco smoke. The primary risk factor for COPD of those who smoke, about 20% will get COPD, and of those who are lifelong smokers, about half will get COPD. For the same amount of cigarette smoking, women have a higher susceptible risk of COPD than men (34). Additionally, the likelihood of developing COPD increases with secondhand smoke exposure (Figure 2). Typically, these must occur over several decades before symptoms develop. A person's genetic makeup also affects the risk. Environmental factors contribute to the development of COPD, with occupational exposure and pollution from indoor fires being significant causes in some countries, and there is convincing evidence that smoking may alter individual susceptibility (35). COPD is a heterogeneous collection of diseases with different causes, pathogenic mechanisms, and physiological effects. COPD is caused by cigarette smoking and is the third greatest cause of mortality in the United States. In the United States and United Kingdom, of those with COPD, 80–95% are either current smokers or previously smoked. In non-smokers, exposure to SHS exposure is the cause in up to 20% of cases. COPD is associated with sustained inflammation, excessive injury, and accelerated lung aging (36). Chronic inflammation is a recognized pathogenic mechanism underlying COPD. Lung obstruction cannot be cured, but it is a common chronic disease that can be prevented and treated (37). According to estimates by the World Health Organization, the prevalence of global population is around 5%. Morbidity and mortality are currently the third leading cause of death in the United States (38). Most of the COPD seen in men, with a high prevalence and a chronic course, especially tobacco use and indoor air pollution (such as heating biofuels), patients with frequent and long-term adjuvant oxygen therapy or medication (Figure 2). Therefore, establishing a correct diagnosis of COPD and appropriate symptom relief treatment, especially dyspnea and prolonging survival are the main problems facing medical science. Smoking is a major cause of human chronic obstructive pulmonary disease (COPD) (39). However, the mechanism by which nicotine induces the COPD remains obscure, although in nicotine carcinogenesis, promotion co-carcinogenesis may have crucial roles. Nicotine, cigarette smoke extract, exhibits COPD and promoting activities in tumor production (40). All reports evidence, nicotine promoted COPD in all patients, the role of nicotine underlying mechanisms through α7nAChR nicotine receptor signaling in lung cancer is still unknown. To determine nicotine induces COPD cell lines proliferation, cell growth, and migration using immunoblot and immunofluorescent analysis.

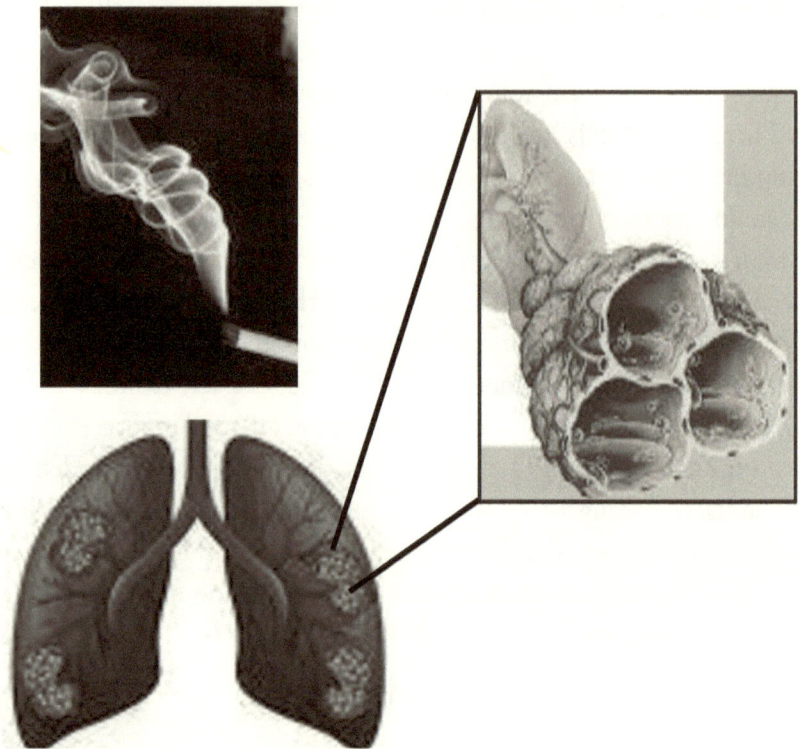

Figure 2. Chronic Obstructive Pulmonary Disease (COPD), known as lung obstruction, is a common respiratory disease characterized by persistent expiratory flow. Lung obstruction can not be cured, but it is a common chronic disease that can be prevented and treated. Most of the COPD seen in men, with a high prevalence and a chronic course, especially tobacco use and indoor air pollution (such as secondhand smoke exposure), patients with frequent and long-term adjuvant oxygen therapy or medication.

1.4. SHS Exposure Induces Lung Cancer

Cigarette carcinogens on the HDAC2-related signaling in lung cancer cells, cigarette smoke extract will be freshly produced by the following indicated methodology. Notably, SHS is used to check if our clinical observations come mainly from nicotine. HDAC2 expression plasmid will be transiently transfected into lung cancer cells for designed time points and doses. Meanwhile, SHS and/or nicotine at different doses and time points will be co-treated to determine the modulations of HDAC2 on nicotine-mediated bio-effects. Cancer can start almost is a condition in which cells in a particular part of the body grow out of control and reproduce. Normal human cells grow and divide to form new cells. Cancer cell differs from normal cells; one difference is that cancer cells grow out of control, no mature specific functions and become invasive, continue to divide without stopping (41). To determine effects of HDAC2 on nicotine-mediated bio-effects in cell cycle fraction, indirect immunofluorescent staining, Brd and rH2AX labeling test to determine S phase cells and DNA damage response, wound healing assay to determine effects of HDAC2 on nicotine-mediated migration ability of SCLC cells, and *in vitro* invasion assay to determine effects of HDAC2 on nicotine-mediated invasion activity. Short-term cisplatin treatment at different doses within one to seven days will be also applied using the same methods to determine the modulations of HDAC2 as well as its interplay with nicotine on cisplatin-mediated bio-effects. It should be noted that all our findings above will be confirmed by specific approach. Normal cells mature into specific function cell types as the body needs. When human cells have grown, new cells take their place. When cells grown old or become damaged, they die. Cancer cells grow and divide uncontrollably but do not respond appropriately to signals that control the normal behavior of cells. Cancer cells can invade and destroy healthy tissues around, including organs (42). Benign tumors do not spread into nearby tissue. Cancerous tumors are malignant. These tumors grow and travel to distant places in the body. Sometimes malignant cancer develops in one part of the body and then spreads to other parts of the body, a process known as metastasis. There are currently over 200 different types of cancer, each of which has its own diagnostic and therapeutic approach. Cancer is a genetic disease, damage DNA caused from environmental exposures (43), such as Chemicals or tobacco smoke. Non-small cell lung cancer is the most common type of lung cancer. About 85% of lung cancers are non-small cell lung cancers. Squamous cell carcinoma, adenocarcinoma, and large cell carcinoma are all subtypes of non-small cell lung cancer (44). Small cell lung cancer is also called oat cell cancer. They are sometimes called lung neuroendocrine tumors. Most of these tumors grow slowly and rarely spread (45). Cancer begins to some of the body's cells during their divide without stopping in all types of organs and then spread into surrounding tissues. When cells grown old and become damaged may be able to influence the normal cells. Cancer cells may be able to influence the normal cells. Blood vessels supported tumors with oxygen and nutrients leading to growth and feed, maybe induced normal cells from cancer cells (46).

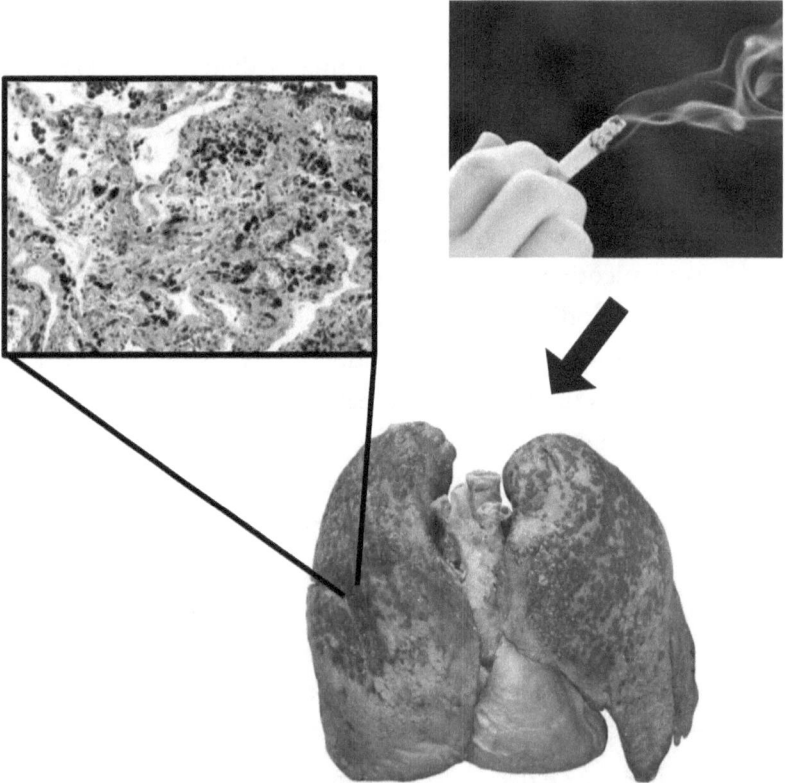

Figure 3. Smoking activates cancer cell different from normal cells. In normal cells, growth requires a balance between the activity of those

genes that promote cell proliferation. Smoking relies on the activities of damaged genes signal to cancerous.

On the other hand, blood vessels also remove waste products from tumors. Tumors can also use the immune system to stay alive and grow. Cancer is causing a unique combination of genetic changes with environmental exposures such as the chemicals in tobacco smoke or radiation. Different cells may have different genetic changes (46-47). The immune system in normal removes damaged or abnormal cells from the body, however, cancer cells will be able to "hide" from the immune system. Cancer is a gene disease caused by certain changes to genetic or inheritance (Figure 3). Benign tumors removed, they usually don't grow back, but malignant were not (48). Benign tumors do not spread and invade into nearby tissues. However, brain benign brain can be life-threatening. Even though the same tumor in different cells may have different genetic changes. Cancer cells have mutations in DNA than normal cells. Cancer cell tends to three main types of genes: proto-oncogenes, tumor suppressor genes, and DNA repair genes (49). Proto-oncogenes are involved in normal cell growth and division. However, when these genes are altered in certain ways or are more active than normal, they may become cancer-causing genes (or oncogenes), allowing cells to grow and survive when they should not. Cancer is causing a unique combination of genetic changes with environmental exposures, such as the chemicals in tobacco smoke or radiation (Figure 3). Cancer begins to some of the body's cells during their divide without stopping in all type of organ and then spread into surrounding tissues. Sometimes malignant cancer develops in one part of the body and then spreads to other parts of the body, a process known as metastasis (50). There are currently over 200 different types of cancer, each of which has its own diagnostic and therapeutic approach. Cancer is a genetic disease, damages DNA caused by environmental exposures, such as Chemicals or tobacco smoke. More than 1.2 million people die of lung cancer each year. Lung cancer is also the first frequently diagnosed cancer in Taiwan, and it accounts for 20% of cancer deaths.

The major patients of lung cancer are non-small cell lung cancer (NSCLC), which comprises approximately 80% of all new lung cancer patients. Non-small cell lung cancer is the most common type of lung cancer. Almost all lung cancers are non-small cell lung cancers including squamous cell carcinoma, adenocarcinoma, and large cell carcinoma are all subtype of non-small cell lung cancer (51). About 10%~15% of lung cancers are small-cell lung cancer. This type of lung cancer tends to spread quickly. Lung Carcinoid Tumor is fewer than 5% of lung cancers. They are also sometimes called lung neuroendocrine tumors. Most of these tumors grow slowly and rarely spread (52). Despite the large number of clinical trials aimed at improving patient survival, lung cancer remains a leading cause of cancer-related mortality worldwide in both men and women. Notably, lung adenocarcinoma, the predominant histological subtype of NSCLC, accounts for 20-30% of primary lung cancer cases among subjects under 45 years of age, regardless of smoking history (53). Lung cancer is caused by environmental exposures, such as the tobacco smoke. Lung cancer is also the first frequently diagnosed cancer, and it accounts for 20% of cancer deaths. The major patients of lung cancer are non-small cell lung cancer (NSCLC), which comprises approximately 80% of all new lung cancer patients. Non-small cell lung cancer is the most common type of lung cancer (54). There is currently malignant cancer developing in one part of the body and then spreading to other parts of the body, a process known as metastasis, each of which has its own diagnostic and therapeutic approach (55). They are also sometimes called lung neuroendocrine tumors. Each stage of the host response is under genetic control. More than a million people die of non-small cell lung cancer each year. Non-small cell lung cancer is one type of lung cancer. Lung cancer develops to grow out of control to become abnormal. Malignant lung cancers are always found contain both small cell lung carcinoma (SCLC) and non-small cell lung cancer (NSCLC) (56). The majority of adenocarcinoma is found in smokers' lung cancer. A history of tobacco smoking is a more common squamous cell carcinoma of the lung. However, NSCLC is usually not very sensitive to chemotherapy and radiation. The NSCLC patient can typically be classified three different categories: (i) Early/non-metastatic disease patients (stage I, II, and III tumors). (ii) Late/locally advanced disease confined large tumors, tumors involving critical chest structures or positive mediastinal lymph nodes to the thoracic cavity. (iii). Patients with cancer cells distant metastasis outside of the thoracic cavity. At an early stage, a small and inoperable tumor may undergo high-intensity radiation (57). However, NSCLC is usually not very sensitive to chemotherapy and radiation. Tobacco smoking which lead to DNA damage. SHS exposure contains more than six thousand components. Smoking is the leading risk factor for lung cancer (58). Secondhand smoke exposure or air pollution appears to be the primary underlying cause of cancer. DNA damage from cigarette smoke is the cause of NSCLC. NSCLC is leading many forms of deficiencies in DNA repair. Incomplete repair leads to damages increase. DNA damage from SHS exposure is the cause of NSCLC. Incomplete repair lead to damages increase. We found that nicotine was able to increase the NO production through inducing nitric oxide synthase 2 (NOS2) expressions and HDAC2 which was upon nicotine (59). Cancer development is not restricted to genetic changes but may also involve epigenetic changes. The main epigenetic modifications in mammals, and particularly in humans, are DNA methylation and posttranslational histone modifications (60).

Histone deacetylases enzymes (HDAC) is an enzyme to lead to histone chemical modification after translation. The acetylation of histones level controlled post-translation modification and epigenetic gene regulation. HDAC2 plays a circle role in cancer cells' physiological roles including development and growth, depending on the specific extracellular environment. Lung cancers with the chemotherapy-resistant phenotype (61). Chemotherapy drugs and target drugs may be recommended. Chemotherapy drugs, these types of drugs interfere with the way cells work and can kill cells in various phases of the cell cycle. These drugs may be combined to attack cancer cells in different ways (62). Most cases of NSCLC are unsuitable for surgery and chemotherapy remains the cornerstone of treatment for advanced disease.

Platinum-based doublet chemotherapy remains the mainstay for advanced NSCLC, but toxicities including leukopenia, nephrotoxicity, or neurotoxicity hinder its application (63). Although EGFR tyrosine kinase inhibitor leads to a great treatment advance of NSCLC, only a subgroup with EGFR activating mutation benefits from it. Hence, the development of new anti-lung cancer drugs or treatments has become an important and urgent issue. Chemotherapy drugs target cells at different phases of the process of forming the cell cycle (64). Chemotherapy is a kind of drug that kills cancer cells to treat tumors. The main function of these drugs is to inhibit the different parts of the tumor cell cycle. Depending on the effect of the drug on cell proliferation kinetics, drugs that differentiate cell cycle-specific and cell cycle non-specific tumors. Target drugs as a form of molecular medicine targeted therapy blocks the growth of cancer cells by interfering with specific targeted molecules needed for carcinogenesis and tumor growth (65), rather than by simply interfering with all rapidly dividing cells. Antibody-drug conjugates combine biologic and cytotoxic mechanisms into one targeted therapy. A drug therapy that blocks the growth of cancer cells by interfering with the specific molecules required for canceration or tumor proliferation. Targeted therapy can reverse the malignant phenotype of tumor cells (66). Not all cancer patients are eligible for targeted therapy. Targeted therapy may be limited to patients whose tumor site has the proper target for a targeted therapeutic drug to play a role (67). Sometimes a patient is eligible for a targeted therapy only if the patient meets certain conditions (for example, cancer does not respond to other therapies, cancer has spread, or can't be surgically removed (68). Cancer development is not restricted to genetic changes but may also involve epigenetic changes. The main epigenetic modifications in mammals, and particularly in humans, are DNA methylation and posttranslational histone modifications (69). Several mechanisms account for the cisplatin-resistant of tumor cells that have been described. First, the action of cisplatin underlies the anticancer potential. Cisplatin is intracellularly spontaneously activated in the cytoplasm by a low concentration of Chloride ions resulted in the generation of mono- and bi-cisplatin forms. In the cytoplasmic, cisplatin has the potential to deplete reduced equivalents and to destroy the redox balance toward oxidative stress (70). And cancer cell is also susceptible to inactivation by a number of cytoprotective antioxidant systems. Cisplatin inserts and binds DNA tightly caused by a predilection for nucleophilic N7-sites on purine bases (71). Therefore, we discuss and provide some conclusions the mechanisms about the cisplatin effects as following: (a) steps process the binding of cisplatin to DNA (72), (b) binding direct relative to DNA and cisplatin adducts (73), (c) concerning the cisplatin mediated DNA damage lethal signaling pathway (74). (d) affecting off-target resistance molecular circuitries do not present obvious links with cisplatin-elicited signals (75). As in some clinical settings, cisplatin constitutes the major therapeutic option, the development of chemosensitization strategies constitutes a goal with important clinical implications (76). We detected the best-characterized mode of action of cisplatin involves the DNA-damage response and mitochondrial apoptosis. Cisplatin involves the DNA-damage response is time- and dose-dependent. The molecular mechanisms account for the cisplatin-resistant phenotype (77). Peptide leukotriene receptor antagonists may be recommended. Cysteinyl leukotriene receptor antagonist (CysLTR) drugs, these types of drugs interfere with the way cells work and can kill cells in various phases of the cell cycle. These drugs may be combined to attack cancer cells in different ways. The CysLT1 receptor antagonist drugs target cells at different phases of the process of forming the cell cycle (78). Cysteinyl leukotriene receptor antagonists are a kind of drug that kills cancer cells to treat tumors. The main function of these drugs is to inhibit the different parts of the tumor cell cycle. Depending on the effect of the drug on cell proliferation kinetics, drugs that differentiate cell cycle-specific and cell cycle non-specific tumors. CysLTR drugs as a form of molecular medicine targeted therapy blocks the growth of cancer cells by interfering with specific targeted molecules needed for carcinogenesis and tumor growth (79), rather than by simply interfering with all rapidly diving cells. Cysteinyl leukotriene receptor antagonists drug conjugates combine biologic and cytotoxic mechanisms into one therapy. Cysteinyl leukotriene receptor antagonist (CysLTR) drugs therapy that blocks the growth of cancer cells by interfering with the specific molecules required for canceration or tumor proliferation. Cysteinyl leukotriene receptor antagonist (CysLTR) drugs therapy can reverse the malignant phenotype of tumor cells (80). Not all cancer patients are eligible for Cysteinyl leukotriene receptor antagonist (CysLTR) drugs therapy. Cysteinyl leukotriene receptor antagonist (CysLTR) drugs therapy may be limited to patients whose tumor site has the proper for therapeutic drugs to play a role (81). Cysteinyl leukotriene receptor antagonists (LTRAs) such as montelukast and zafirlukast have been recently reported to protect asthma patients from developing cancers, especially lung cancers. Zafirlukast is a synthetic peptide leukotriene receptor antagonist (LTRA). Zafirlukast is an oral leukotriene receptor antagonist (LTRA) for asthma, usually dosed twice daily (82). Zafirlukast blocks the action of the cysteinyl leukotrienes on the CysLT1 receptors, reducing inflammation of the breathing passages in the lungs. On the other hand, leukotriene receptor antagonists (LTRAs) with mild side effects, have anti-metastatic activity in epidermoid carcinoma, lung carcinoma, and colon cancers as well as neuroprotective effects. LTRAs inhibited migration and invasion of cancer cell, and cysteinyl leukotriene receptor 1 (CysLT1) play a role in human carcinogenesis (83). Because of favorable safety profile and beneficial anti-inflammatory properties, the CysLT1 receptor antagonists (LTRA), zafirlukast, approved for the treatment of asthma and are frequently prescribed as add-on therapeutics to reduce the amount of inhaled glucocorticoids and $\beta2$-agonists (84). Thus, the role of leukotrienes in antimicrobial defenses, cancer, cardiovascular disease, and asthma is mentioned. The blockade of leukotriene synthesis and leukotriene receptors is explored. CysLTs in cell culture or animal models of inflammation and cancer have to be reassessed carefully if higher doses of LTRA were applied or serum levels in cell culture assays were low (85). These results implicated that cysteinyl leukotriene receptor 1 (CysLT1) might be required for carcinogenic content-mediated advanced development or zafirlukast treatment failure in lung cancer (86). Intriguingly, this association seen in the CysLT1 receptor antagonist groups was demonstrated in only squamous cell lung cancer (SC) but not in adenocarcinoma (AD), providing the specific interplay between CysLT1 receptor antagonists and carcinogenic content of cysteinyl leukotriene receptor 1 (87). It has been demonstrated that the CysLT1 receptor might have tumor-promoting or co-carcinogenic activity. Treatment with CysLT1 receptor antagonists, zafirlukast, induced the NO production through rapidly increasing NOS2 expression, and subsequently was nitrosylated. To access effects of acute and chronic exposure of SHS and/or nicotine, we will also establish SHS- and nicotine-tolerant cell lines in lung cancer cells. These cell lines will be also analyzed via XTT assay, FACS analysis, indirect immunofluorescent staining, wound healing assay, and *in vitro* invasion assay, and angiogenesis assay. In addition, the effects of HDAC2 stably overexpressing cells on SHS- or nicotine-mediated effects will be also examined. After comparison of short-term and long-term examinations, we may find the universal and unique characteristics of HDAC2 on nicotine-mediated effects. To determine downstream signaling at translation levels, real-time PCR to determine downstream signaling at transcription levels, subcellular fractionation assay to examine subcellular localization of HDAC2 related signaling effectors, chromatin immunoprecipitation to confirm transcriptional regulation of HDAC2 for downstream signaling, and immunoprecipitation to examine potential protein-protein interaction of HDAC2 with other transcription factors, depending on step by step experimental results and demand, will be used for further exploration of downstream signaling (88). Nicotine signaling will be also analyzed together by the mentioned approaches. The knockdown of CysLT1 receptor reduced CysLT1 induced inflammation. Treatment with zafirlukast may be enhanced the cytotoxicity of inhibited invasion ability in both H226, H2170, H520, and H1703 (SCLC) cells, suggesting that zafirlukast may increase therapeutic resistance effects of zafirlukast-based treatments and therefore has potential to be applied in the clinic to improve patient survival of NSCLC (Figure 4). It is important to disclose such common proteins exerting pleiotropic effects on lung cancer because we may be able to identify the individuals of zafirlukast with the poor outcomes with lung cancer (89). Therefore, appropriate zafirlukast treatment can be taken far earlier lung cancer develops. In this project, we try to identify the roles and underlying mechanisms of NO with a focus on its interplay with zafirlukast potentially resulted in therapy resistance in lung cancer cells (90). We aim to develop treatment strategies for the interplay of NOS with zafirlukast and potentially resulted in therapy resistance and/or metastasis in *vitro* and in *vivo* (Figure 4). Therefore, we have three major goals to accomplish in this project. Sometimes a patient is eligible for a targeted therapy only if the patient meets certain conditions (for example, cancer does not respond to other therapies, cancer has spread, or cannot be surgically removed) (91). Cysteinyl leukotriene receptor 1 and CysLT1 receptor antagonists are targeted drugs. Zafirlukast can bind to cysteinyl leukotriene receptor 1 on the surface of tumor cells with mutations to inhibit cysteinyl leukotriene receptor 1 activity of tumor cells (Figure 4), thereby blocking downstream inhibiting tumor function. Zafirlukast is only effective in about 40% of patients with non-small cell lung cancer in Asia before using it for genetic testing (92). The median survival for patients with mutations in the cysteinyl leukotriene receptor. Indications in non-small cell lung cancer, especially lung adenocarcinoma. Zafirlukast's mechanism of action is similar to that of CysLT1 receptor antagonists, which can bind to the CysLT1 receptor with a mutation that blocks the tumor cells (93). Only about 40% of Asian patients with non-small cell lung cancer effective. The aim of this study was to explore the mechanisms of combined zafirlukast's in lung cancer development and death. We suggest combination strategies may be exploited for reverting cisplatin resistance in tumors. Histone deacetylases (HDAC) modulates acetylation of lysine residues, the formation of the core histone complex (H2A, H2B, H3, and H4) plays a critical role to regulate cell cycle progression and cell developmental associated transcription factor, YY1, a zinc-finger protein (94). They may have additional independent roles in human physiologic functions and cancer cells. Zafirlukast's was dispensable for HDAC1 binding to HDAC2-activated targets, zafirlukast's was required for the recruitment of HDAC1 to repressed HDAC2 gene. The role of nicotine through HDAC in lung cancer growth. Nicotine constitutes approximately 0.6-3.0% of the dry weight of tobacco. Like anything that enters the body, nicotine is also metabolized. Therefore, any activity that increases your metabolic rate can help speed up the clearance of nicotine (95). Exercise is a good way to increase the rate of metabolism. Exercise improves heart rate and increases the rate of metabolism and burning of heat. For people who have many years of smoking, it is important to start exercising. Make sure to drink plenty of water because nicotine is soluble in water, so drinking water helps to excrete the substance through the urine. Vitamin A is also helpful in removing nicotine from the body because it also has the effect of speeding up the metabolism. Because nicotine tends to destroy vitamin C in the body, it is important to supplement it after quitting smoking (96).

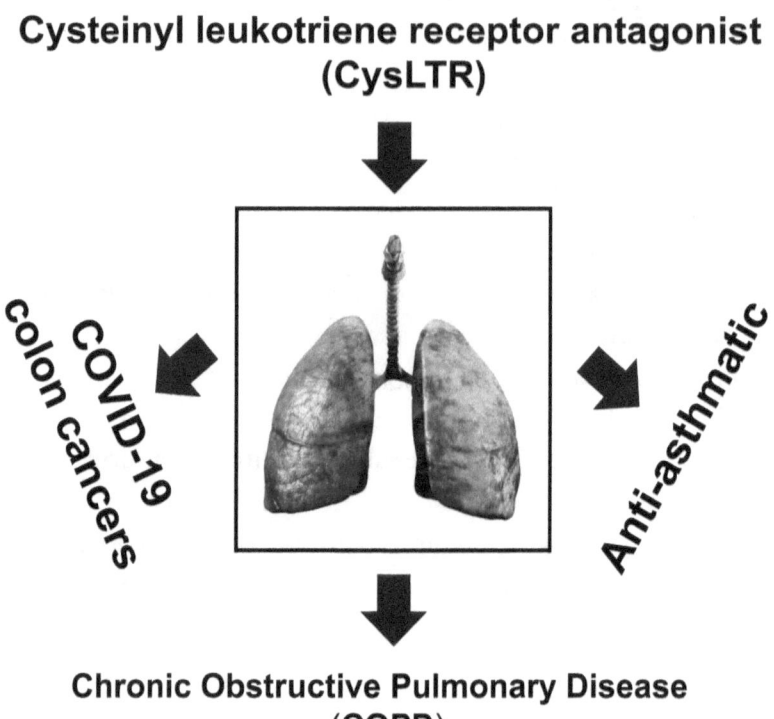

Figure 4. Zafirlukast, a Cysteinyl leukotriene receptor antagonist (CysLTR), can reduce short-acting asthma, COPD, and lung cancer, improving the lung function.

1.5. Lung Cancer

Sometimes malignant cancer develops in one part of the body, then spreads to other parts of the body, a process known as metastasis. There are currently over 200 different types of cancer, each of which has its own diagnostic and therapeutic approach. Cancer is a genetic disease, damage DNA caused from environmental exposures, such as the chemicals or tobacco smoke. More than 1.2 million people die of lung cancer each year (97). The major patients of lung cancer are non-small cell lung cancer (NSCLC), which comprises approximately all new lung cancer patients. Non-small cell lung cancer is the most common type of lung cancer. Lung cancers are non-small cell lung cancers. Squamous cell carcinoma, adenocarcinoma and large cell carcinoma are all subtype of non-small cell lung cancer. Small cell lung cancer is also called oat cell cancer. About 10%~15% of lung cancers are small cell lung cancer. This type of lung cancer tends to spread quickly. Lung carcinoid tumor is fewer of lung cancers. They are also sometimes called lung neuroendocrine tumors. Most of these tumors grow slowly and rarely spread (98). Despite of the large number of clinical trials aimed at improving patient survival, lung cancer remains a leading cause of cancer-related mortality worldwide in both men and women. Notably, lung adenocarcinoma, the predominant histological subtype of NSCLC, regardless of smoking history. However, our evidences reported nicotine induces NOS2 and γ-H2AX expression levels in transfect HDAC2 into H157 lung cancer cells. HDAC2 siRNA significantly downregulated the expression of HDAC2 proteins in H157 cells. Nicotine proliferation lung cancer cells and resistance cell cycle arrest mediated by regulated HDAC2 expression increased may be tightly associated with the increase of cyclin D1, cyclin D2, cyclin D3, cyclin E, cyclin B1, CDK4, and cdc25c protein expression (99). In nuclear could observed p-HDAC2 increased and PARP decreased. Location of HDAC2 protein expression levels in nuclear, cytosol and nuclear plus cytosol. Long-term nicotine 24 h and 48 h induced, cell-cycle-related protein expression and anti-apoptosis at 48 h was higher than 24 h in H157 cell lines. Nicotine leads to VPA and cisplatin loose its functions in H520 cell line. And nicotine let to H520 cell viability higher and HDAC2 protein expression in nuclear increases. Nicotine increases migration and invasion of lung cancer cells through activation of the α7nAChR. It is suggested that the effects of NNK appear to be mostly dependent upon the α7nAChR. HDAC2 frequency, implicating that HDAC2 might be required for cigarette carcinogenic content-mediated advanced development or treatment failure in total lung cancer cases, regardless of tissue types. Intriguingly, this association seen in smoker and non-smoker groups was demonstrated in only squamous cell carcinoma (SC), but not in adenocarcinoma (AD), confirming the specific interplay between HDAC2 and carcinogenic content of cigarette. It is that the contribution of increased HDAC2 to a poor survival rate is limited in those smokers with SC lung cancer. On the other hand, those associations seen in relapse and relapse-free patients were observed in all lung cancer cases, despite of tissue types, suggesting the critical role of HDAC2 in treatment failure/resistance or metastasis of lung cancer. Treatment with valporic acid (VPA), a HDAC2-specific inhibitor, significantly increased the cytotoxicity of cisplatin in both A549 (AD) and H520 (SC) cells. Hence, aberrant interplay of HDAC2 with nicotine may be required for its oncogenic activity in SC lung cancer, and HDAC2 may be required for treatment failure/resistance or metastasis and therefore contributes to relapse (100). It is important to disclose such a common protein exerting pleiotropic effects on lung cancer because we may be able to identify the individuals with poor outcome in lung cancer patients. In addition, appropriate treatment and prevention can be taken far earlier after/before lung cancer develops. Therefore, we have four major goals to accomplish in this project. This is a very first study linking nicotine to HDAC2 aberrations in lung cancer. Notably, nicotine constitutes approximately 0.6–3.0% of the dry weight of tobacco. The accomplishment of this project will not only provide better understanding of lung cancer development but also provide useful information for the clinicians to decide the appropriate drugs/treatments for each individual lung cancer patient. Our findings suggested that aberrations of HDAC2 may play some critical roles in NSCLC. Thus, with the accomplishment of this project, we may develop more effective treatment strategy for lung cancer using clinically available HDAC2 inhibitor such as valporic acid (101). Establish H157N long-term nicotine treatment for more than one-year model. Immunofluorescence assay of HDAC2 proteins in H157 cells treated with nicotine (1 µM) for time-dependent and/or pretreated. Immunofluorescence assay of HDAC2 proteins in H157N cells treated with long-term nicotine treatment for more than one year (1 µM) for time-dependent and/or pretreated. Immunoblot analysis of H157 cells treated with nicotine (1 µM) and HDAC2 transfection (wt).

Cell lyses were immunoblotted with the proteins for p-HDAC2, NOS2, p-AKT, AKT, and β-actin antibodies. Immunoblot analysis of γ-H2AX, H2AX, p-chk2, chk2, Bcl-2, and Mcl-1 in H157 and H157 cells upon a long-term treatment with nicotine. HDAC2: HDAC2 small interfering (si)RNA, VPA: valporic acid. Knockdown of HDAC2 (Si) abolished nicotine-induced invasive activity. Treatment with valporic acid (VPA), a HDAC2-specific inhibitor, significantly enhanced inhibitory effects of cisplatin on invasion ability and enhanced the cytotoxicity of cisplatin in H157 (SC) cells. Inhibition of HDAC2 activity (si HDAC2) may increase relative chk-2 suppressed tumor gene and inhibition Bcl-2 and Mcl-1 protein expression. Cisplatin-based treatments. Therefore, has potential to be applied in clinic to improve patient survival of NSCLC. One histone post-translational modifications associated with DNA damage repair is gamma histone H2AX (γ-H2AX). Cisplatin-promoted rH2AX in H157 cells decreased those in A549 cells. Precancerous lesions of the lung were found to contain signs of a DNA damage response, which included the presence of histone H2AX. These distinct effects seemed to be dependent on tissue types and required further investigations. H157 cells upon a long-term treatment with nicotine. Immunoblot analysis of H157 cells treated with nicotine (1 μM). Immunofluorescence assay of HDAC2 proteins in H157N cells treated with long-term nicotine treatment for more than one year (1 μM) for time-dependent and/or pretreated. Immunoblot analysis of H157 and H157 transfect HDAC2 cells treated with nicotine time-dependent (1 μM). Immunoblot analysis of H157 and H157 treated with nicotine (1 μM) time-dependent transfect HDAC2 cells. H157N (long-term nicotine treatment for more than one year) and H157 treatment nicotine long-term in cell membrane related mechanisms. Immunofluorescence assay of p-HDAC2, NOS2, sanil, ZO-1, TCF8/ZEB1, vimentin, N-cadherin, claudin-1, γ-H2AX proteins in H157N (cells treated with long-term nicotine treatment for more than one year) (1 μM). H157 treatment nicotine long-term in cell membrane related mechanisms. Long-term nicotine at 24h and 48 h relative cell cycle and cell apoptosis in H157 and H520 cell line. Protein expression using western blotting.

HDAC2 expression level location in H157 cell line. H520 cell viability using MTT analysis. HDAC2 in nuclear location expression in nicotine H520 cell line. Nicotine potently induces phosphorylation of cell-cycle-related protein expression via activation of different time, which is associated with accelerated migration of human lung cancer cells. It is noted that HDAC2 is one of transcription factor responsible for metastasis of H520 and H520 plus nicotine. Likewise, combined loss of HDAC2 was linked to de-repression of γ-H2AX and Bax in the lung. Accordingly, proliferating cells cannot tolerate simultaneous lack of HDAC2, implying that cisplatin drugs and VPA inhibiting both enzymes are promising anti-cancer drugs. Compared with H157 and H520 cell treated with nicotine, cell apoptosis protein mechanism using western blotting. Nicotine suppression apoptosis signaling related protein such as c-jun, c-fos, stat1, and stat3. H520 tumor growth and proliferation related mechanisms. time-dependent nicotine treatment in cell cycle by western blot. migration of H520 human lung cancer cells. Cell cycle and proliferation related protein in H520 and H520 plus nicotine. H157 and H520 cell growth signaling in cytosol and in nuclear. Cell growth related protein in H157 and H520 cell line exposure nicotine. Immunofluorescence assay showed that HDAC2 enhanced in H520 and in H157 cells in nuclear. H520 and H520 plus nicotine cell line in cell growth signaling in cytosol and in nuclear. Nicotine and HDAC2 transfection increased H520 cell growth higher than H157 cell line. Nicotine rapidly increased production of nuclear of HDAC2 from immunoprecipitation results showed. Nicotine increased transfection rate of H520 and H157, when HDAC2 was ectopically overexpressed. Upon nicotine treatment, nuclear HDAC2 will be rapidly shuttled to the cytoplasm determined and immunofluorescence assay, suggesting his nicotine-mediated trans-localization may be involved in its modulation of HDAC2 activity (101). Carcinogens form the link between nicotine addiction and lung cancer, and DNA adducts are crucial in this process. Cancer development is not restricted to the genetic changes but may also involve epigenetic changes (75). The main epigenetic modifications in mammals, and particularly in humans, are

DNA methylation and posttranslational histone modifications (46). More recent studies indicate, however, that additional deleterious effects of nicotine might be mediated through cell-surface receptors. Nicotine binds to nicotinic-acetylcholine receptors (nAChRs) and other receptors, leading to activation of the serine/threonine kinase Akt (protein kinase B), protein kinase A, and other factors. This leads to downstream effects, such as decreased apoptosis, increased cell proliferation, and transformation. Nicotine also stimulates angiogenesis and tumor growth, which is also mediated through nAChRs, possibly involving endothelial production of nitric oxide (NO), prostacyclin, and vascular endothelial growth factor. These data indicate that nicotine might have tumor-promoting or co-carcinogenic activity.

1.6. The Role of Nicotine through HDAC Induces Lung Cancer Growth

SHS exposure is highly addictive. Smoking exposure is insufficient as a carcinogen, it functions as a tumor promoter on purpose. It follows that nicotine is associated with cancer in humans. SHS exposure also promotes cancer growth, angiogenesis, and neovascularization. Thereby, smoking exposure impeding apoptosis, promoting tumor growth and activating growth factors. Smoking exposure binds to nicotinic-acetylcholine receptors (nAChR) or EGF receptors, leading to activation of protein kinase B, protein kinase A, and other factors (97). This leads to downstream effects, such as decreased apoptosis, increased cell proliferation and transformation. Smoking exposure also stimulates angiogenesis and tumor growth which is also mediated through nicotinic-acetylcholine receptors (nAChR), possibly involving endothelial production of nitric oxide (NO), prostacyclin and vascular endothelial growth factor (98). We found that smoking exposure was able to increase the NO production through inducing nitric oxide synthase 2 (NOS2) expressions and HDAC2 which was nitrosylated upon smoking exposure treatment and further reduced by L-NAME, a NOS inhibitor. Various solid tumors including gastric, colon, cervical cancers, and endometrial stromal sarcomas have an obviously increased HDAC2 expression. Consistently, HDAC2 depletion causes growth arrest and apoptosis of certain human cancer cells. Several observations can explain these findings. For example, HDAC2 represses INPP5F and GSK3β/APC-mediated degradation of β-catenin, which supports the link between HDAC2 expression and tumor development. In addition, HDAC2 inhibits the tumor suppressor p53 and promotes MYC expression (99). This can establish vicious circles that hamper apoptosis and cell cycle arrest. The following table illustrates distinct targets and functions in different cell types or organs. Histone H2AX phosphorylation on a serine four residues from the carboxyl terminus (producing γH2AX) is a sensitive marker for DNA double-strand breaks (DSBs). DSBs may lead to cancer but, paradoxically, are also used to kill cancer cells (100). Using γH2AX detection to determine the extent of DSB induction may help detect precancerous cells to stage cancers, to monitor the effectiveness of cancer therapies and to develop novel anticancer drugs. During the tobacco curing and smoking process, smoking exposure can be converted to mainly 4-(methylnitrosamino)-1-(3-pyridyl)-1-butanone (NNK) through nitrosation. In SC, NNK-induced proliferation appears to involve activation of the α7nAChR, MEK, protein kinase C (PKC), and c-myc. Repeated exposure of SC to smoking exposure increases collagen breakdown and transmigration in conjunction with increased tumor growth, vascularity, and resistance to chemotherapy (101). SHS exposure increases migration and invasion of lung cancer cells through activation of the α7nAChR. It is suggested that the effects of NNK appear to be mostly dependent upon the α7nAChR. The modification of the structure of these N-terminal tails of histones by acetylation/deacetylation is crucial in modulating gene expression. Besides, lysine acetylation of histones is reversible and histone deacetylases (HDACs) play a critical role in reversing histone hyperacetylation (102). Except for the histones, the HDACs also have many non-histone proteins substrates, which regulate cell proliferation and cell death. Accumulating evidence has pointed out the increased expression of HDAC2 in several solid tumors including gastric, colon, cervical cancers, and endometrial stromal sarcomas. However, its role in lung cancer remains to be largely lacking (103). In this project, we try to identify the interplay of HDAC2 with cigarette carcinogens (*i.e.,* nicotine) and potentially resulted in treatment resistance (*i.e.,* cisplatin) NSCLC in particular squamous cell carcinoma (SC). In addition, we aim to develop corresponsive treatment strategies (104). Histone deacetylases enzymes (HDAC2) is an enzyme to lead to histone chemical modification after translation. The acetylation of histones level controlled post-translation modification gene regulation. To detect HDAC activity maybe for developing HDAC drugs. HDAC2 plays a circle role in cancer cells' physiological roles including development and differentiation, depending on the specific environment (105). Histone acetylation activates chromatin acetylation that leads to transcriptional activation; in contrast, deacetylation of histone leads to chromatin structures condensed suppressing gene expression (106). Therefore, the inhibition of HDACs causes transcription activation of cancer-suppressor genes, such as cyclin-dependent kinase inhibitor p21, resulting in cell-cycle arrest and apoptosis induction in malignant cells. Histone deacetylases (HDAC) modulates acetylation of lysine residues; the formation of the core histone complex plays a critical role to regulate cell cycle progression and cell developmental associated transcription factor, YY1, a zinc-finger protein. They may have additional independent roles in human physiologic functions and cancer cells (107). Nicotine constitutes approximately of tobacco. Like anything that enters the body, nicotine is also metabolized. Therefore, any activity that increases your metabolic rate help speed up the clearance of nicotine. Thereby, smoking exposure impeding apoptosis, promoting tumor growth and activating growth factors. Consistently, HDAC2 depletion causes growth arrest and apoptosis of certain human cancer cells. Several observations can explain these findings (108). In addition, HDAC2 inhibits the tumor suppressor p53 and promotes MYC expression. This can establish vicious circles that hamper apoptosis and cell cycle arrest. The following table illustrates distinct targets and functions in different cell types or organs. Histone H2AX phosphorylation on serine four residues from the carboxyl terminus (producing γH2AX) is a sensitive marker for DNA double-strand breaks (DSBs). DSBs may lead to cancer but, paradoxically, are also used to kill cancer cells (109). Using γH2AX detection to determine the extent of DSB induction may help detect precancerous cells, to stage cancers, to monitor the effectiveness of cancer therapies and to develop novel anticancer drugs. Histone deacetylases enzymes (HDAC2) is an enzyme to lead to histone chemical modification after translation (110). The acetylation of histones level controlled post-translation modification and epigenetic gene regulation. To detect HDAC activity maybe for developing HDAC-targeting drugs. HDAC2 plays a circle role in normal and cancer cells physiological roles including development and differentiation, depending on the specific tissue and extracellular environment. Histone acetylation activates chromatin acetylation lead to transcriptional activation, in contrast, deacetylation of histone lead to chromatin structures condensed suppressing gene expression (111). Therefore, the inhibition of HDACs cause transcription activation of cancer-suppressor genes, such as cyclin-dependent kinase inhibitor p21, resulting in cell-cycle arrest and apoptosis induction in malignant cells. Histone deacetylases (HDAC) modulates acetylation of lysine residue, the formation of the core histone complex (H2A, H2B, H3, and H4) plays a crucial role to regulate cell cycle progression and cell developmental associated transcription factor, YY1, a zinc-finger protein. They may have additional independent roles in human physiologic functions and cancer cells (112). HDAC2 was dispensable for HDAC1 binding to HDAC2-activated targets; HDAC2 was required for the recruitment of HDAC1 to repressed HDAC2 gene. Histone H2AX phosphorylation on a serine four residues from the carboxyl terminus (producing γH2AX) is a sensitive marker for DNA double-strand breaks (DSBs). DSBs may lead to cancer but, paradoxically, are also used to kill cancer cells (113). Using γH2AX detection to determine the extent of DSB induction may help to detect precancerous cells, to stage cancers, to monitor the effectiveness of cancer therapies and to develop novel anticancer drugs (114). Inhibition of HDACs led to cell cycle arrest at G1/S phase by alteration of cell cycle regulatory proteins. Cell growth inhibition and apoptosis may be a result of HDAC2-mediated cyclin D1 suppression. Down-regulation of HDAC2 expression mediates proliferation inhibition and cell cycle arrest. It is associated with a decrease in cyclin D1, cyclin E, and CDK2 protein expression and an increase in p21 protein expression (115). Constitutively, expressed NOS isoforms are activated by calmodulin via an increase of intracellular calcium concentration. Considering iNOS-derived NO as a multifactorial transmitter of tumorigenesis and tumor progression (116). Blood pressure regulation, inflammation, infection, and the onset and progression of malignant diseases. The role of nicotine and α7nAchR in lung cancer growth. It is suggested that the effects of nicotine appear to be mostly dependent upon the α7nAChR. Nicotine is the leading risk factor of lung cancer (117). The nAChRs are complex structures composed of five transmembrane subunits arranged. This leads to the downregulation effects of cell growth as well as decreased apoptosis, increased cell proliferation, and transformation. Although nicotine is not a carcinogen, it may influence cancer development and progression or effectiveness of anti-cancer therapy (118). Stimulating the receptors in the cancer cells leads to downstream activation of multiple signaling cascades that promote cancer cell survival, proliferation, angiogenesis, migration, and metastasis in a tumor-specific manner. Several trials have evaluated the influence of nicotine on lung cancer cells (119). The mechanisms by which nicotine impacts cancer biology involve suppression of apoptosis induced by certain drugs or radiation promotion of proliferation, angiogenesis, invasion, and migration of cancer cells (120). This effect is mainly mediated by membranous nicotinic acetylcholine receptors whose stimulation leads to sustained activation of such intracellular pathways as PI3K/Akt/mTOR, RAS/RAF/MEK/ERK and induction of NF-κB activity enhanced transcription of mitogenic promoters, inhibition of the mitochondrial death pathway or stimulation of pro-angiogenic factors (121). The mechanisms underlying nicotine's influence on the biology of lung cancer cells and the effectiveness of anti-cancer therapy. Protein expression levels of α7nAChR, NOS2 and cell cycle related proteins were examined. Primary results showed nicotine promotedα7nAChR, NOS2 and cell cycle-related protein, Cyclin D1/pRb, and Cyclin E/E2F, increases. Therefore, we suggest nicotine promoted cell cycle actives through receptor α7nAChR induced. In the previous study, we also want to know nicotine related to cell cytoplasm and nuclear regulation. Nicotine increases the migration and invasion of lung cancer cells through activation of the α7nAChR (122). Nicotine binds to nicotinic-acetylcholine receptors (α7nAchR) and other receptors, leading to activation of the Akt, PI3K and other factors. Nicotine directly regulated NOS2 expression in an α7nAchR dependent manner. Its activation resulted in the regression of tumor cell growth and inactivation of cellular apoptosis via DNA damage to α7nAchR α activation in H157 lung cancer cells (123). A time-dependent nicotine treatment-induced NOS2 expression and p-Akt increases. Because the frequent loss of function of the NOS2 protein by nitrosylation was reported in lung cancer, the nicotine-mediated induction of NOS2 may provide one of its links to α7nAchR (124). On the other hand, NSCLC cells included adenocarcinoma and squamous lung cancer cells. They are different functions between adenocarcinoma and squamous. Smoker or nicotine exposure may affect either adenocarcinoma or squamous (125). In this study, we determine nicotine induced squamous cancer cells proliferation and cell growth but not adenocarcinoma cancer cells. This control is still unclear until today. Furthermore, we detected cell membrane receptor proteins, α7nAChR related-nicotine effects. This effects maybe is time-dependent and dose-dependent to regulate NSCLC cell growth (126). That is our anticipated results and want to resolution. Intricately, we can use these findings to help new drugs development. To detect HDAC activity maybe for developing HDAC-targeting drugs. HDAC2 plays a circle role in normal and cancer cells physiological roles including development and differentiation, depending on the specific tissue and extracellular environment. Histone acetylation activates chromatin acetylation lead to transcriptional activation, in contrast, deacetylation of histone lead to chromatin structures condensed suppressing gene expression. Therefore, the inhibition of HDACs causes transcription activation of cancer-suppressor genes, such as cyclin-dependent kinase inhibitor p21, resulting in cell-cycle arrest and apoptosis induction in malignant cells. Histone deacetylases (HDAC) modulates acetylation of lysine residues, formation of the core histone complex (H2A, H2B, H3 and H4) plays a critical role to regulate cell cycle progression and cell developmental associated transcription factor, YY1, a zinc-finger protein. They may have additional independent roles in human physiologic functions and cancer cells. HDAC2 was dispensable for HDAC1 binding to HDAC2-activated targets, HDAC2 was required for the recruitment of HDAC1 to repressed HDAC2 gene. Nicotine constitutes approximately 0.6~3.0% of the dry weight of tobacco. Like anything that enters the body, nicotine is also metabolized. Therefore, any activity that increases your metabolic rate can help speed up the clearance of nicotine. Exercise is a good way to increase the rate of metabolism. Exercise improves heart rate and increases the rate of metabolism and burning of heat. For people who have many years of smoking, it is important to start exercising. Make sure to drink plenty of water because nicotine is soluble in water, so drinking water helps to excrete the substance through the urine (127). Vitamin A is also helpful in removing nicotine from the body because it also has the effect of speeding up the metabolism. Because nicotine tends to destroy vitamin C in the body, it is important to supplement it after quitting smoking. Nicotine is highly addictive. Nicotine is insufficient as a carcinogen, it's functions as a tumor promoter on purpose. It follows that nicotine is associated with cancer in humans. Nicotine also promotes cancer growth, angiogenesis and neovascularization. Thereby, nicotine impeding apoptosis, promoting tumor growth and activating growth factors. Nicotine binds to nicotinic-acetylcholine receptors (nAChR) or EGF receptors, leading to activation of protein kinase B, protein kinase A, and other factors. This leads to downstream effects, such as decreased apoptosis, increased cell proliferation and transformation. Nicotine also stimulates angiogenesis and tumor growth which is also mediated through nicotinic-acetylcholine receptors (nAChR), possibly involving endothelial production of nitric oxide (NO), prostacyclin and vascular endothelial growth factor. We found that nicotine was able to increase the NO production through inducing nitric oxide synthase 2 (NOS2) expressions and HDAC2 which was nitrosylated upon nicotine treatment, and further reduced by L-NAME, a NOS inhibitor. Various solid tumors including gastric, colon, cervical cancers, and endometrial stromal sarcomas have an obviously increased HDAC2 expression (128). Consistently, HDAC2 depletion causes growth arrest and apoptosis of certain human cancer cells. Several observations can explain these findings. For example, HDAC2 represses INPP5F and GSK3β/APC-mediated degradation of β-catenin, which supports the link between HDAC2 expression and tumor development. In addition, HDAC2 inhibits the tumor suppressor p53 and promotes MYC expression. This can establish vicious circles that hamper apoptosis and cell cycle arrest. The following table illustrates distinct targets and functions in different cell types or organs. Histone H2AX phosphorylation on a serine four residues from the carboxyl terminus (producing γH2AX) is a sensitive marker for DNA double-strand breaks (DSBs). DSBs may lead to cancer but, paradoxically, are also used to kill cancer cells. Using γH2AX detection to determine the extent of DSB induction may help to detect precancerous cells, to stage cancers, to monitor the effectiveness of cancer therapies and to develop novel anticancer drugs. During the tobacco curing and smoking process, nicotine can be converted to mainly 4-(methylnitrosamino)-1-(3-pyridyl)-1-butanone (NNK) through nitrosation. In SC, NNK-induced proliferation appears to involve activation of the α7nAChR, MEK, protein kinase C (PKC), and c-myc. Repeated exposure of SC to nicotine increases collagen breakdown and transmigration in conjunction with increased tumor growth, vascularity, and resistance to chemotherapy. The aberrant regulation of HDAC2 and its epigenetic regulation of gene transcription in apoptosis and cell cycle components are suggested to play an important role in lung cancer development. We found a positive HDAC2 staining was mainly observed in the nucleus of squamous lung cancer cells as expected. To explore the potential roles of HDAC2 protein in lung cancer, the immunohistochemistry was firstly used to analyze the distribution patterns of HDAC2 protein in NSCLC. Treatment with nicotine did not significantly change the levels of total HDAC2 proteins in cytoplasm. However, upon nicotine treatment, nuclear HDAC2 will be rapidly shuttled to the cytoplasm into nuclear was determined and immunofluorescence assay, suggesting this nicotine-mediated trans-localization may be involved in its modulation of HDAC2 activity. We also established the H520N (long-term nicotine treatment for more than one year) and found that HDAC2 proteins were increased in cytoplasmic fraction. HDAC2 directly regulated NOS2 expression in a HDAC2-dependent manner. Its activation resulted in regression of tumor cell growth and inactivation of cellular apoptosis *via* DNA damage and Bax suppression and Bcl-2 activation in H157 lung cancer cells. A time-dependent nicotine treatment induced NOS2 expression and p-Akt increases. Because frequent loss of function of the HDAC2 protein by nitrosylation was reported in neurons, the nicotine-mediated induction of NOS2 may provide one of its links to HDAC2. In addition, sustained-suppression of HDAC2 in H157 lung cancer cells attenuated in vitro tumorigenic properties tumor growth. Taken together, these studies suggest that aberrant HDAC2 expression may be involved in advanced lung cancer development. Cigarette smoke has been shown to cause DNA damage and to impair double-strand break (DSB) repair, which is aggravated in patients with COPD/emphysema. A recent study has demonstrated that HDAC2 functions in the DNA damage response (DDR) along with HDAC1 to promote DNA repair. Long-term nicotine treatment did not have any obvious induction of NOS2. HDAC2 regulates chromatin plasticity and enhances DNA vulnerability. This may be caused by HDAC2-mediated transcriptional repression, which prevents transcription from interfering with the repair process. Another possibility is that HDAC2 recruitment influences the ability of DNA repair factors. HDAC2 bind the damaged DNA and function effectively. In addition, HDAC1 and HDAC2 was found to affect the persistence of nicotine factors at DSBs resulted in hypersensitivity to DNA-damaging agents suggesting a function of these enzymes in the DDR, such as NOS2, α7nAchR, CKIIα, Histone-H3. Zonula occludens-1 (ZO-1) is well known as tight junction protein-1. This gene encodes a protein located on a cytoplasmic membrane surface of intercellular tight junctions. This encoded protein may be involved in signal transduction at cell and cell junctions (129). The protein encoded by this gene, including TCF/ZEB1, N-cadherin and claudin-1 in epithelial or endothelial cell sheets. Vimentin has a significant role to attached to offering flexibility to the cell. Because of vimentin supports the anchoring position to dynamic attached the nucleus, endoplasmic reticulum, and mitochondria to the organelles in the cytosol. Therefore, HDAC2 transfection and cisplatin did not have significantly different changes in vimentin protein expression. The because vimentin is responsible for maintaining cell shape, integrity of the cytoplasm, and stabilizing cytoskeletal interactions.

1.7. Lung Cancer with Chemotherapy-Resistant Phenotype

Chemotherapy drugs and target drugs may be recommended. Chemotherapy drugs, these types of drugs interfere with the way cells work and can kill cells in various phases of the cell cycle. These drugs may be combined to attack cancer cells in different ways. Most cases of NSCLC are unsuitable for surgery and chemotherapy remains the cornerstone of treatment for advanced disease. Platinum-based doublet chemotherapy remains the mainstay for advanced NSCLC, but toxicities including leukopenia, nephrotoxicity, or neurotoxicity hinder its application (12). Although EGFR tyrosine kinase inhibitor leads to a great treatment advance of NSCLC, only a subgroup with EGFR activating mutation benefits from it. Hence, the development of new anti-lung cancer drugs or treatments has become an important and urgent issue. Chemotherapy drugs target cells at different phases of the process of forming the cell cycle (130). Chemotherapy is a kind of drugs that kill cancer cells to treat tumors. The main function of these drugs is to inhibit the different parts of the tumor cell cycle.

Depending on the effect of the drug on cell proliferation kinetics, drugs that differentiate cell cycle specific and cell cycle non-specific tumors. Target drugs as a form of molecular medicine, targeted therapy blocks the growth of cancer cells by interfering with specific targeted molecules needed for carcinogenesis and tumor growth (11), rather than by simply interfering with all rapidly dividing cells. Antibody-drug conjugates combine biologic and cytotoxic mechanisms into one targeted therapy (22). A drug therapy that blocks the growth of cancer cells by interfering with the specific molecules required for canceration or tumor proliferation. Targeted therapy can reverse the malignant phenotype of tumor cells (131). Not all cancer patients are eligible for targeted therapy. Targeted therapy may be limited to patients whose tumor site has the proper target for a targeted therapeutic drug to play a role (64). Sometimes, a patient is eligible for targeted therapy only if the patient meets certain conditions (for example, the cancer does not respond to other therapies, the cancer has spread, or can not be surgically removed). Cancer development is not restricted to the genetic changes, but may also involve epigenetic changes. The main epigenetic modifications in mammals, and particularly in humans, are DNA methylation and posttranslational histone modifications (35). The modification of the structure of these N-terminal tails of histones by acetylation/deacetylation is crucial in modulating gene expression. Besides, lysine acetylation of histones is reversible and histone deacetylases (HDACs) play a critical role in reversing histone hyperacetylation (16). Except from the histones, the HDACs also have many non-histone proteins substrates, which regulate cell proliferation and cell death. Accumulating all evidences have pointed out increased expression of HDAC2 in several solid tumors including gastric, colon, cervical cancers, and endometrial stromal sarcomas (132). However, its role in lung cancer remains to be largely lacking. In this project, we try to identify the interplay of HDAC2 with cigarette carcinogens (*i.e.,* nicotine) and potentially resulted treatment resistance (*i.e.,* cisplatin) in NSCLC in particular squamous cell carcinoma (SC). In addition, we aim to develop corresponsive treatment strategies *in vitro* and in *vivo*

(118). Histone deacetylases enzymes (HDAC2) is an enzyme to lead to histone chemical modification after translation. The acetylation of histones level controlled post-translation modification and epigenetic gene regulation (133).

Our results had shown that treatment with VPA significantly attenuated the cytotoxicity of cisplatin in both A549 and H520 cells. Although HDAC2 cannot directly or independently predict patient survival, HDAC2 appeared to be required for advanced SC lung cancer development mediated by carcinogenic content of cigarette smoke and for treatment failure or resistance in NSCLC.

Conclusion

Therefore, combinational treatments with drugs targeting HDAC2, such as VPA, Quisinostat, or CUDC-907, may provide benefits to improve patient survival in NSCLC. A549, H520, H520N, H157, and stably overexpressing HDAC2 clones, as well as cisplatin-resistant cell clone, which have been established in specific (134). Furthermore, HDAC2 expression plasmid or siRNA (shRNA plasmid) will be transiently transfected into lung cancer cells for designed time points and doses determined in Aim 2 to examine the effects of combinational treatments with cisplatin and other HDAC2 inhibitors. XTT assay (to determine effects of treatments alone or in combination), FACS analysis (to determine cell cycle fraction), indirect immunofluorescent staining (Brdu and γH2AX labeling test to determine S phase cells and DNA damage response), wound healing assay (to determine effects of treatments alone or in combination), and *in vitro* invasion assay (determine effects of treatments alone or in combination). HDAC2 expression plasmid will be transiently transfected into A549 (AD), H520 (SC), and H157 (SC) cells and the immortalized lung fibroblast, HFL-1, for different time points and doses. A549 cells and HFL-1 cells serve as a control for checking if our observations are tissue-specific effect and if nicotine action in the very early stage or advanced stage. We have also harvested a H520 cell lines/clones for more than one-year nicotine treatment (named H520N). H157 and other cells will be harvested at the same condition. If necessary, HDAC2 mutants will be construed depending on clinical observations and/or experimental results. For example, we will establish nucleus- or cytoplasm-localized HDAC2 mutant if we need to examine HDAC2 function when trans-localized to different subcellular spaces. Nicotine, nicotine inhibitors, HDAC2 inhibitors, and/or cisplatin will treat these cells alone or in combination. As for long-term effects, the lung cancer cell line, stably overexpressing HDAC2 (*i.e.*, HDAC2 stable clone), will be constructed. In addition, we will also establish cisplatin-resistant cell lines allowing us to confirm effects of HDAC2 on cisplatin resistance in lung cancer cells (135). To develop treatment strategies for the interplay HDAC2 with nicotine as well as potentially resulted in Cisplatin treatment failure/resistance in NSCLC cells. HDAC2-specific activators, such as Theophyline, will be used to compare or confirm our observations (136). Theophylline is a bronchodilator at high doses, that possibly due to an effect on increase of HDAC2 activity, resulting in suppression of inflammatory genes and enhancement of the anti-inflammatory effects of glucocorticoids. In addition, Sulforaphane has been suggested to be able to restore HDAC2 activity in the alveolar macrophages and lungs of mice exposed to CSE. Thus, we will use *in vitro* system first with different drug combinations to find the curative strategy to treat NSCLC, including SC lung cancer. Furthermore, DDR-related signaling (BRCA1, p53, CBP, γH2AX, H3K56, and Ku70), HDAC2-mediated signaling (*e.g.* p21, Rb1, BMP4, and NF-κB), anti-apoptotic (Bcl-2 family members) and pro-apoptotic proteins (PUMP, caspase family and PARP) will be analyzed together (137). As for cell cycle distribution, FACS analysis will be first used to analyze, while immunoblotting approach will be used to analyze the levels of cell cycle-specific cyclins (*e.g.* cyclin D, E, and A/B), cyclin-dependent kinases (cdk 2, cdk4, cdk6, and cdc2), and checkpoint proteins (chk1 and chk2).

References

1. Cantalupo, P. G.; Katz, J. P.; Pipas, J. M. *Viral Sequences in Human Cancer.* Virology. 2017;513:208-16.

2. Reedijk, A. M. J.; Van der Heiden-Van der Loo, M.; Visser, O.; Karim-Kos, H. E.; Lieverst, J. A.; De Ridder-Sluiter, J. G.; Coebergh, J. W. W.; Kremer, L. C.; Pieters, R. *Site of Childhood Cancer Care in the Netherlands.* Eur J Cancer. 2017;87: 38-46.

3. Shin, V. Y.; Liu, E. S.; Ye, Y. N.; Koo, M. W.; Chu, K. M.; Cho, C. H. *A Mechanistic Study of Cigarette Smoke and Cyclooxygenase-2 on Proliferation of Gastric Cancer Cells.* Toxicol Appl Pharmacol. 2004;195:103-12.

4. Yang, T.; Chang, P. Y.; Park, S. L.; Bastani, D.; Chang, S. C.; Morgenstern, H.; Tashkin, D. P.; Mao, J. T.; Papp, J. C.; Rao, J. Y.; Cozen, W.; Mack, T. M.; Greenland, S.; Zhang, Z. F. *Tobacco Smoking, NBS1 Polymorphisms, and Survival in Lung and Upper Aerodigestive Tract Cancers with Semi-Bayes Adjustment for Hazard Ratio Variation.* Cancer Causes Control. 2014;25:11-23.

5. Ward, M.; Norman, H.; D'Souza, M. S. *Effects of Pharmacological Manipulation of the Kappa Opioid Receptors on the Aversive Effects of Nicotine.* Behav Brain Res. 2017;338:56-65.

6. Sanner, T.; Grimsrud, T. K. *Nicotine: Carcinogenicity and Effects on Response to Cancer Treatment - A Review.* Front Oncol. 2015;5:196.

7. Zhang, J.; Kamdar, O.; Le, W.; Rosen, G. D.; Upadhyay, D. *Nicotine Induces Resistance to Chemotherapy by Modulating Mitochondrial Signaling in Lung Cancer.* Am J Respir Cell Mol Biol. 2009;40:135-46.

8. Riggare, S.; Unruh, K. T.; Sturr, J.; Domingos, J.; Stamford, J. A.; Svenningsson, P.; Hägglund, M. *Patient-Driven N-of-1 in Parkinson's Disease. Lessons Learned from a Placebo-Controlled Study of the Effect of Nicotine on Dyskinesia.* Methods Inf Med. 2017;56:e123-e128.

9. Grozio, A.; Catassi, A.; Cavalieri, Z.; Paleari, L.; Cesario, A.; Russo, P. *Nicotine, Lung, and Cancer.* Anticancer Agents Med Chem. 2007;7:461-6.

10. Xu, T.; Li, D.; Wang, H.; Zheng, T.; Wang, G.; Xin, Y. *MUC1 Downregulation Inhibits Non-Small Cell Lung Cancer Progression in Human Cell Lines.* Exp Ther Med. 2017;14:4443-7.

11. Williams, R. S.; Williams, J. S.; Tainer, J. A. *Mre11-Rad50-Nbs1 Is a Keystone Complex Connecting DNA Repair Machinery, Double-Strand Break Signaling, and the Chromatin Template.* Biochem Cell Biol. 2007;85:509-20.

12. Puig-Vilanova, E.; Martínez-Llorens, J.; Ausin, P.; Roca, J.; Gea, J.; Barreiro, E. *Quadriceps Muscle Weakness and Atrophy Are Associated with a Differential Epigenetic Profile in Advanced COPD.* Clin Sci (Lond). 2015;128:905-21.

13. Frenzel, T.; Hoffmann, B.; Schmitz, R.; Bethge, A.; Schumacher, U.; Wedemann, G. *Radiotherapy and Chemotherapy Change Vessel*

Tree Geometry and Metastatic Spread in a Small Cell Lung Cancer Xenograft Mouse Tumor Model. PLoS One. 2017;12:e0187144.

14. Yamaguchi, M.; Hirai, F.; Taguchi, K.; Toyozawa, R.; Edagawa, M.; Shimamatsu, S.; Nosaki, K.; Seto, T.; Takenoyama, M.; Ichinose, Y. *A Typical Carcinoid Tumor of the Lung Presenting with Pure Persistent Ground-Glass Opacity on High-Resolution Computed Tomography: A Case Report.* Surg Case Rep. 2017;3: 108.

15. Zhang, X.; Li, D.; Wang, H.; Pang, C.; Wu, Y.; Wen, F. *Gender Difference in Plasma Fatty-Acid-Binding Protein 4 Levels in Patients with Chronic Obstructive Pulmonary Disease.* Biosci Rep. 2016;36:e00302.

16. Samareh Fekri, M.; Torabi, M.; Azizi Shoul, S.; Mirzaee, M. *Prevalence and Predictors Associated with Severe Pulmonary Hypertension in COPD.* Am J Emerg Med. 2018;36:277-80.

17. Jensen, K. P.; DeVito, E. E.; Sofuoglu, M. *How Intravenous Nicotine Administration in Smokers Can Inform Tobacco Regulatory Science.* Tob Regul Sci. 2016; 2:452-63.

18. Esrick, E. B.; McConkey, M.; Lin, K.; Frisbee, A.; Ebert, B. L. *Inactivation of HDAC1 or HDAC2 Induces Gamma Globin Expression without Altering Cell Cycle or Proliferation.* Am J Hematol. 2015;90:624-28.

19. Fan, Y.; Wang, K. *Nicotine Induces EP4 Receptor Expression in Lung Carcinoma Cells by Acting on AP-2α: The Intersection between Cholinergic and Prostanoid Signaling.* Oncotarget. 2017;8:75854-63.

20. Yang, Y.; Deng, Y.; Chen, X.; Zhang, J.; Chen, Y.; Li, H.; Wu, Q.; Yang, Z.; Zhang, L.; Liu, B. *Inhibition of PDGFR by CP-673451 Induces Apoptosis and Increases Cisplatin Cytotoxicity in NSCLC*

Cells via Inhibiting the Nrf2-Mediated Defense Mechanism. Toxicol Lett. 2018;295:88-98.

21. Zeng, F.; Li, Y. C.; Chen, G.; Zhang, Y. K.; Wang, Y. K.; Zhou, S. Q.; Ma, L. N.; Zhou, J. H.; Huang, Y. Y.; Zhu, W. Y.; Liu, X. G. *Nicotine Inhibits Cisplatin-Induced Apoptosis in NCI-H446 Cells.* Med Oncol. 2012;29:364-73.

22. Warren, G. W.; Singh, A. K. *Nicotine and Lung Cancer.* J Carcinog. 2013;12:1.

23. Argentin, G.; Cicchetti, R. *Evidence for the Role of Nitric Oxide in Antiapoptotic and Genotoxic Effect of Nicotine on Human Gingival Fibroblasts.* Apoptosis. 2006.11:1887-97.

24. Sapalidis, K.; Zarogoulidis, P.; Pavlidis, E.; Laskou, S.; Katsaounis, A.; Koulouris, C.; Giannakidis, D.; Mantalovas, S.; Huang, H.; Bai, C.; Wen, Y.; Wang, L.; Sardeli, C.; Amaniti, A.; Karapantzos, I.; Karapantzou, C.; Hohenforst-Schmidt, W.; Konstantinou, F.; Kesisoglou, I.; Benhanseen, N. *Aerosol Immunotherapy with or without Cisplatin for Metastatic Lung Cancer Non-Small Cell Lung Cancer Disease: In vivo Study. A More Efficient Combination.* J Cancer. 2018;9:1973-77.

25. Riley, C. M.; Sciurba, F. C. *Diagnosis and Outpatient Management of Chronic Obstructive Pulmonary Disease: A Review.* JAMA 2019;321:786-97.

26. Ke, J.; Dong, N.; Wang, L.; Li, Y.; Dasgupta, C.; Zhang, L.; Xiao, D. *Role of DNA Methylation in Perinatal Nicotine-Induced Development of Heart Ischemia-Sensitive Phenotype in Rat Offspring.* Oncotarget. 2017;8:76865-80.

27. Grill, S.; Yahiaoui-Doktor, M.; Dukatz, R.; Lammert, J.; Ullrich, M.; Engel, C.; Pfeifer, K.; Basrai, M.; Siniatchkin, M.; Schmidt,

T.; Weisser, B.; Rhiem, K.; Ditsch, N.; Schmutzler, R.; Bischoff, S. C.; Halle, M.; Kiechle, M. *Smoking and Physical Inactivity Increase Cancer Prevalence in BRCA-1 and BRCA-2 Mutation Carriers: Results from a Retrospective Observational Analysis.* Arch Gynecol Obstet. 2017;296:1135-44.

28. Yao, X.; Panichpisal, K.; Kurtzman, N.; Nugent, K. *Cisplatin Nephrotoxicity: A Review.* Am J Med Sci. 2007:334:115-24.

29. Togashi, Y.; Hayashi, H.; Okamoto, K.; Fumita, S.; Terashima, M.; De Velasco, M. A.; Sakai, K.; Fujita, Y.; Tomida, S.; Nakagawa, K.; Nishio, K. *Chronic Nicotine Exposure Mediates Resistance to EGFR-TKI in EGFR-Mutated Lung Cancer via an EGFR Signal.* Lung Cancer. 2015;88:16-23.

30. Bordas, A.; Cedillo, J. L.; Arnalich, F.; Esteban-Rodriguez, I.; Guerra-Pastrián, L.; De Castro, J.; Martín-Sánchez, C.; Atienza, G.; Fernández-Capitan, C.; Rios, J. J.; *Montiel C. Expression Patterns for Nicotinic Acetylcholine Receptor Sub-Unit Genes in Smoking-Related Lung Cancers.* Oncotarget. 2017;8:67878-90.

31. Macqueen, D. A.; Heckman, B. W.; Blank, M. D.; Janse Van Rensburg, K.; Park, J. Y.; Drobes, D. J.; Evans, D. E. *Variation in the α 5 Nicotinic Acetylcholine Receptor Sub-Unit Gene Predicts Cigarette Smoking Intensity as a Function of Nicotine Content.* Pharmacogenomics J. 2014;14:70-6.

32. Schiller, J. H.; Harrington, D.; Belani, C. P.; Langer, C.; Sandler, A.; Krook, J.; Zhu, J.; Johnson, D. H. *Comparison of Four Chemotherapy Regimens for Advanced Non-Small-Cell Lung Cancer.* N Engl J Med. 2002;346:92-8.

33. Wang, H.; Gomez, D. R.; Liao, Z. *β-Blockers and Metastasis in Non-Small-Cell Lung Cancer.* Expert Rev Anticancer Ther. 2013;13:641-3.

34. Faillace, M. P.; Zwiller, J.; Bernabeu, R. O. *Effects of Combined Nicotine and Fluoxetine Treatment on Adult Hippocampal Neurogenesis and Conditioned Place Preference*. Neuroscience. 2015;300:104-15.

35. Afghahi, A.; Sledge, G. W. Jr. *Targeted Therapy for Cancer in the Genomic Era*. Cancer J. 2015;21:294-8.

36. Tsimberidou, A. M. *Targeted Therapy in Cancer*. Cancer Chemother Pharmacol. 2015;76:1113-32.

37. Yang, W.; Gao, Y.; Li, X.; Zhang, J.; Liu, T.; Feng, X.; Pan, H.; Yang, X.; Xie, S.; Feng, X.; Lv, Z.; Wang, Y.; Chen, Z; He, J. *Postoperative Survival of EGFR-TKI-Targeted Therapy in Non-Small Cell Lung Cancer Patients with EGFR 19 or 21 Mutations: A Retrospective Study*. World J Surg Oncol. 2017;15:197.

38. Gonzalez, V. M.; Fuertes, M. A.; Alonso, C. Perez, J. M. *Is Cisplatin-Induced Cell Death Always Produced by Apoptosis?* Mol Pharmacol. 2001;59:657-63.

39. Xu, J.; Huang, H.; Pan, C.; Zhang, B.; Liu, X.; Zhang, L. *Nicotine Inhibits Apoptosis Induced by Cisplatin in Human Oral Cancer Cells*. Int J Oral Maxillofac Surg. 2007;36:739-44.

40. Busch, M.; Papior, D.; Stephan, H.; Dünker, N. *Characterization of Etoposide- and Cisplatin-Chemoresistant Retinoblastoma Cell Lines*. Oncol Rep. 2018;39: 160-172.

41. Cruz-Bermúdez, A.; Vicente-Blanco, R. J.; Laza-Briviesca, R.; García-Grande, A.; Laine-Menéndez, S.; Gutiérrez, L.; Calvo, V.; Romero, A.; Martín-Acosta, P.; García, J. M.; Provencio, M. *PGC-1alpha Levels Correlate with Survival in Patients with Stage 3 NSCLC and May Define a New Biomarker to Metabolism-Targeted Therapy*. Sci Rep. 2017;7:16661.

42. Chatterjee, P. K.; Yeboah, M. M.; Solanki, M. H.; Kumar, G.; Xue, X.; Pavlov, V. A.; Al-Abed, Y.; Metz, C. N. *Activation of the Cholinergic Anti-Inflammatory Pathway by GTS-21 Attenuates Cisplatin-Induced Acute Kidney Injury in Mice.* PLoS One. 2017;12:e0188797.

43. Wang, C.; Niu, W.; Chen, H.; Shi, N.; He, D.; Zhang, M.; Ge, L. Tian, Z.; Qi, M.; Chen, T.; Tang, X. *Nicotine Suppresses Apoptosis by Regulating α7nAChR/Prx1 Axis in Oral Precancerous Lesions.* Oncotarget. 2017;8:75065-75.

44. Cagini, L.; Balloni, S.; Ludovini, V.; Andolfi, M.; Matricardi, A.; Potenza, R.; Vannucci, J.; Siggillino, A.; Tofanetti, F. R.; Bellezza, G.; Bodo, M.; Puma, F.; Marinucci, L. *Variations in Gene Expression of Lung Macromolecules after Induction Chemotherapy for Lung Cancer.* Eur J Cardiothorac Surg. 2017;52:1077-1082.

45. Serrano, E.; Lasa, A.; Perea, G.; Carnicer, M. J.; Brunet, S.; Aventín, A.; Sierra, J.; Nomdedéu, J. F. *Acute Myeloid Leukemia Subgroups Identified by Pathway-Restricted Gene Expression Signatures.* Acta Haematol. 2006;116:77-89.

46. Damia, G.; Filiberti, L.; Vikhanskaya, F.; Carrassa, L.; Taya, Y.; D'incalci, M.; Broggini, M. *Cisplatinum and Taxol Induce Different Patterns of p53 Phosphorylation.* Neoplasia. 2001;3:10-6.

47. Ikeguchi, M.; Kaibara, N. *Changes in Survivin Messenger RNA Level During Cisplatin Treatment in Gastric Cancer.* Int J Mol Med. 2001;8:661-6.

48. Ishida, S.; McCormick, F.; Smith-McCune, K.; Hanahan, D. *Enhancing Tumor-Specific Uptake of the Anticancer Drug Cisplatin with a Copper Chelator.* Cancer Cell. 2010;17:574-83.

49. Yu, D.; Qin, Y.; Jun-Qiang, L.; Shun-Lin, G. *CNPY2 Enhances Resistance to Apoptosis Induced by Cisplatin via Activation of NF-κB Pathway in Human Non-Small Cell Lung Cancer.* Biomed Pharmacother. 2018;103:1658-63.

50. Chaney, S. G.; Campbell, S. L.; Bassett, E.; Wu, Y. *Recognition and Processing of Cisplatin- and Oxaliplatin-DNA Adducts.* Crit Rev Oncol Hematol. 2005;53:3-11.

51. Lan, Q.; Shen, M.; Berndt, S. I.; Bonner, M. R.; He, X.; Yeager, M.; Welch, R.; Keohavong, P.; Donahue, M.; Hainaut, P.; Chanock, S. *Smoky Coal Exposure, NBS1 Polymorphisms, p53 Protein Accumulation, and Lung Cancer Risk in Xuan Wei, China.* Lung Cancer. 2005;49:317-23.

52. Karczmarek-Borowska, B.; Filip, A.; Wojcierowski, J.; Smoleń, A.; Pilecka, I.; Jabłonka, A. *Survivin Antiapoptotic Gene Expression as a Prognostic Factor in Non-Small Cell Lung Cancer: In Situ Hybridization Study.* Folia Histochem Cytobiol. 2005;43:237-42.

53. Mandic, A.; Hansson, J.; Linder, S.; Shoshan, M. C. *Cisplatin Induces Endoplasmic Reticulum Stress and Nucleus-Independent Apoptotic Signaling.* J Biol Chem. 2003;278:9100-6.

54. Michaud, W. A.; Nichols, A. C.; Mroz, E. A.; Faquin, W. C.; Clark, J. R.; Begum, S.; Westra, W. H.; Wada, H.; Busse, P. M.; Ellisen, L. W.; Rocco, J. W. *Bcl-2 Blocks Cisplatin-Induced Apoptosis and Predicts Poor Outcome Following Chemoradiation Treatment in Advanced Oropharyngeal Squamous Cell Carcinoma.* Clin Cancer Res. 2009;15:1645-54.

55. Nishimoto, K.; Karayama, M.; Inui, N.; Yasui, H.; Hozumi, H.; Suzuki, Y.; Furuhashi, K.; Fujisawa, T.; Enomoto, N.; Nakamura, Y.; Inami, N.; Matsuura, S.; Kaida, Y.; Matsui, T.; Asada, K.; Matsuda, H.; Fujii, M.; Toyoshima, M.; Imokawa, S.; Suda, T.

Switch Maintenance Therapy with Docetaxel and Bevacizumab after Induction therapy with Cisplatin, Pemetrexed, and Bevacizumab in Advanced Non-Squamous Non-Small Cell Lung Cancer: A Phase 2 Study. Med Oncol. 2018;35:108.

56. Ren, J. H.; He, W. S.; Nong, L.; Zhu, Q. Y.; Hu, K.; Zhang, R. G.; Huang, L. L.; Zhu, F.; Wu, G. *Acquired Cisplatin Resistance in Human Lung Adenocarcinoma Cells is Associated with Enhanced Autophagy.* Cancer Biother Radiopharm. 2010; 25:75-80.

57. Zinellu, A.; Sotgiu, E.; Fois, A. G.; Zinellu, E.; Sotgia, S.; Ena, S.; Mangoni, A. A.; Carru, C.; Pirina, P. *Blood Global DNA Methylation Is Decreased in Non-Severe Chronic Obstructive Pulmonary Disease (COPD) Patients.* Pulmonary Pharmacology and Therapeutics. 2017;46:11-15.

58. Cantalupo, P. G.; Katz, J. P.; Pipas, J. M. Viral Sequences in Human Cancer. Virology. 2017;513:208-216.

59. Medina-Mirapeix, F.; Bernabeu-Mora, R.; Llamazares-Herrán, E.; Sánchez-Martínez, M.; García-Vidal, J. A.; Escolar-Reina, P. *Interobserver Reliability of Peripheral Muscle Strength Tests and Short Physical Performance Battery in Patients with Chronic Obstructive Pulmonary Disease: A Prospective Observational Study.* Archives of Physical Medicine and Rehabilitation. 2016; 97:p2002.

60. Carbone, D. *Smoking and Cancer.* Am J Med. 1992;93:13S-17S.

61. Lee, H.; Park, J. R.; Yang, J.; Kim, E.; Hong, S. H.; Woo, H. M.; Ryu, S. M.; Cho, S. J.; Park, S. M.; Yang, S. R. *Nicotine Inhibits the Proliferation by Upregulation of Nitric Oxide and Increased HDAC1 in Mouse Neural Stem Cells.* In Vitro Cell Dev Biol Anim. 2014;50:731-9.

62. Riggare, S.; Unruh, K. T.; Sturr, J.; Domingos, J.; Stamford, J. A.; Svenningsson, P.;Hägglund, M. *Patient-Driven N-of-1 in Parkinson's Disease. Lessons Learned from a Placebo-Controlled Study of the Effect of Nicotine on Dyskinesia.* Methods Inf Med. 2017;56:e123-e128.

63. Shen, T.; Le, W.; Yee, A.; Kamdar, O.; Hwang, P. H.; Upadhyay, D. *Nicotine Induces Resistance to Chemotherapy in Nasal Epithelial Cancer.* Am J Rhinol Allergy. 2010;24:e73-7.

64. Bando, T.; Fujimura, M.; Kasahara, K.; Ueno, T.; Matsuda, T. *Selective Beta2-Adrenoceptor Agonist Enhances Sensitivity to Cisplatin in Non-Small Cell Lung Cancer Cell Line.* Oncol Rep, 2000;7:49-52.

65. Yamaguchi, M.; Hirai, F.; Taguchi, K.; Toyozawa, R.; Edagawa, M.; Shimamatsu, S.; Nosaki, K.; Seto, T.; Takenoyama, M.; Ichinose, Y. *A Typical Carcinoid Tumor of the Lung Presenting with Pure Persistent Ground-Glass Opacity on High-Resolution Computed Tomography: A Case Report.* Surg Case Rep. 2017;3: 108.

66. Zhou, H.; Kawamura, K.; Yanagihara, H.; Kobayashi, J.; Zhang-Akiyama, Q. M. *NBS1 Is Regulated by Two Kinds of Mechanisms: ATM-Dependent Complex Formation with MRE11 and RAD50 and Cell Cycle-Dependent Degradation of Protein.* J Radiat Res. 201;58:487-494.

67. Hajji, N.; Wallenborg, K.; Vlachos, P.; Nyman, U.; Hermanson, O.; Joseph, B. *Combinatorial Action of the HDAC Inhibitor Trichostatin A and Etoposide Induces Caspase-Mediated AIF-Dependent Apoptotic Cell Death in Non-Small Cell Lung Carcinoma Cells.* Oncogene. 2008;27:3134-44.

68. Caramori, G.; Adcock, I. M.; Casolari, P.; Ito, K.; Jazrawi, E.; Tsaprouni, L.; Villetti, G.; Civelli, M.; Carnini, C.; Chung, K. F.;

Barnes, P. J.; Papi, A. *Unbalanced Oxidant-Induced DNA damage and Repair in COPD: A Link toward Lung Cancer.* Thorax. 2011,66:521-7.

69. Aoshiba, K.; Zhou, F.; Tsuji, T.; Nagai, A. *DNA Damage as a Molecular Link in the Pathogenesis of COPD in Smokers.* Eur Respir J. 2012;39:1368-76.

70. Sun, D. M.; Tang, B. F.; Li, Z. X.; Guo, H. B.; Cheng, J. L.; Song, P. P.; Zhao, X. *MiR-29c Reduces the Cisplatin Resistance of Non-Small Cell Lung Cancer Cells by Negatively Regulating the PI3K/Akt Pathway.* Sci Rep. 2018;8:8007.

71. Banerjee, J.; Al-Wadei, H. A.; Schuller, H. M. *Chronic Nicotine Inhibits the Therapeutic Effects of Gemcitabine on Pancreatic Cancer in Vitro and in Mouse Xenografts.* Eur J Cancer. 2013;49:1152-8.

72. Tsimberidou, A. M. *Targeted Therapy in Cancer.* Cancer Chemother Pharmacol. 2015;76:1113-32.

73. Yang, W.; Gao, Y.; Li, X.; Zhang, J.; Liu, T.; Feng, X.; Pan, H.; Yang, X.; Xie, S.; Feng, X.; Lv, Z.; Wang, Y.; Chen, Z.; He, J. *Postoperative Survival of EGFR-TKI-Targeted Therapy in Non-Small Cell Lung Cancer Patients with EGFR 19 or 21 Mutations: A Retrospective Study.* World J Surg Oncol. 2017;15:197.

74. Busch, M.; Papior, D.; Stephan, H.; Dünker, N. *Characterization of Etoposide- and Cisplatin-Chemoresistant Retinoblastoma Cell Lines.* Oncol Rep. 2018; 39: 160-172.

75. Zhu, W.; Li, Z.; Xiong, L.; Yu, X.; Chen, X.; Lin, Q. *FKBP3 Promotes Proliferation of Non-Small Cell Lung Cancer Cells through Regulating Sp1/HDAC2/p27.* Theranostics. 2017;7:3078-89.

76. Crocetti, E.; Paci, E. *Trends in Lung Adenocarcinoma Incidence and Survival.* Lung Cancer. 2002;35:215-6.

77. Ingadottir, A. R.; Beck, A. M.; Baldwin, C.; Weekes, C. E.; Geirsdottir, O. G.; Ramel, A.; Gislason, T.; Gunnarsdottir, I. *Association of Energy and Protein Intakes with Length of Stay, Readmission, and Mortality in Hospitalized Patients with Chronic Obstructive Pulmonary Disease.* Br J Nutr. 2018;119:543-51.

78. Guo, Q.; Lan, F.; Yan, X.; Xiao, Z.; Wu, Y.; Zhang, Q. *Hypoxia Exposure Induced Cisplatin Resistance Partially via Activating p53 and Hypoxia Inducible Factor-1α in Non-Small Cell Lung Cancer A549 Cells.* Oncol Lett. 2016;16:801-8.

79. Lu, M.; Marsters, S.; Ye, X.; Luis, E.; Gonzalez, L.; Ashkenazi, A. *E-cadherin Couples Death Receptors to the Cytoskeleton to Regulate Apoptosis.* Mol Cell. 2014;54:987-98.

80. Nishioka, T.; Luo, L. Y.; Shen, L.; He, H.; Mariyannis, A.; Dai, W.; Chen, C. *Nicotine Increases the Resistance of Lung Cancer Cells to Cisplatin through Enhancing Bcl-2 Stability.* Br J Cancer. 2014;110:1785-92.

81. Ren, J. H.; He, W. S.; Nong, L.; Zhu, Q Y.; Hu, K.; Zhang, R. G.; Huang, L. L.; Zhu, F.; Wu, G. *Acquired Cisplatin Resistance in Human Lung Adenocarcinoma Cells Is Associated with Enhanced Autophagy.* Cancer Biother Radiopharm. 2010; 25:75-80.

82. Balkan, A.; Bulut, Y.; Fuhrman, C. R.; Fisher, S. N.; Wilson, D. O.; Weissfeld, J. L.; Sciurba, F. C. *COPD Phenotypes in a Lung Cancer Screening Population.* Clin Respir J. 2016;10:48-53.

83. Gabano, E.; Ravera, M.; Zanellato, I.; Tinello, S.; Gallina, A.; Rangone, B.; Gandin, V.; Marzano, C.; Bottone, M. G.; Osella, D. *An Unsymmetric Cisplatin-Based Pt(iv) Derivative Containing*

2-(2-propynyl) Octanoate: A Very Efficient Multi-Action Antitumor Prodrug Candidate. Dalton Trans. 2017;46:14174-85.

84. Fernandez, H. R.; Gadre, S. M.; Tan, M.; Graham, G. T.; Mosaoa, R.; Ongkeko, M. S.; Kim, K. A.; Riggins, R. B.; Parasido, E.; Petrini, I.; Pacini, S.; Cheema, A.; Varghese, R.; Ressom, H. W.; Albanese, C.; Üren, A.; Paige, M.; Giaccone, G.; Avantaggiati, M. L. *The Mitochondrial Citrate Carrier, SLC25A1, Drives Stemness and Therapy Resistance in Non-Small Cell Lung Cancer.* Cell Death Differ. 2018;25:1239-58.

85. Sun, J. M.; Chen, H. Y.; Moniwa, M.; Litchfield, D. W.; Seto, E.; Davie, J. R. *The Transcriptional Repressor Sp3 Is Associated with CK2phosphorylatedhistone Deacetylase 2.* J Biol Chem. 2002;277:35783-6.

86. Li, S.; Wang, F.; Qu, Y.; Chen, X.; Gao, M.; Yang, J.; Zhang, D.; Zhang, N.; Li, W.; Liu, H. *HDAC2 Regulates Cell Proliferation, Cell Cycle Progression and Cell Apoptosis in Esophageal Squamous Cell Carcinoma EC9706 Cells.* Oncol Lett. 2017;13:403-9.

87. Cerosaletti, K.; Concannon, P. *Independent Roles for Nibrin and Mre11-Rad50 in the Activation and Function of Atm.* J Biol Chem 2004;279:38813-9.

88. Gong, T.; Cui, L.; Wang, H.; Wang, H.; Han, N. *Knockdown of KLF5 Suppresses Hypoxia-Induced Resistance to Cisplatin in NSCLC Cells by Regulating HIF-1α-Dependent Glycolysis through Inactivation of the PI3K/Akt/mTOR Pathway.* J Transl Med. 2018;16:164.

89. Borges Rodrigo, C.; Carvalho Celso, R. *Impact of Resistance Training in Chronic Obstructive Pulmonary Disease Patients During Periods of Acute Exacerbation.* Archives of Physical Medicine and Rehabilitation 2014;95:1638.

90. Farooqi, A. A.; Kamran Majeed, S. M.; Mansoor, Q.; Ismail, M. *Population-Specific Genetic Variation at MicroRNA-629-Binding Site in the 3'-UTR of NBS1 Gene in Prostate Cancer Patients.* J Exp Ther Oncol. 2017;11:161-3.

91. Chen, J. H.; Zheng, Y. L.; Xu, C. Q.; Gu, L. Z.; Ding, Z. L.; Qin, L.; Wang Yi; Fu, R.; Wan, Y. F.; Hu, C. P. *Valproic Acid (VPA) Enhances Cisplatin Sensitivity of Non-Small Cell Lung Cancer Cells via HDAC2 Mediated Down Regulation of ABCA1.* Biol Chem, 2017;398:785-92.

92. Gao, W.; Yuan, C.; Zhang, J.; Li, L.; Yu, L.; Wiegman, C. H.; Barnes, P. J.; Adcock, I. M.; Huang, M.; Yao, X. *Klotho Expression Is Reduced in COPD Airway Epithelial cells: Effects on Inflammation and Oxidant Injury.* Clin Sci (Lond). 2015;129:1011-23.

93. Zhu, Y. M.; Gan, Y. L.; Xu, H. Y.; Chen, W. H.; Dai, H. P. *Clinical Effectiveness of Pemetrexed Combined with Cisplatin Chemotherapy for Advanced and Maintenance Treatment for Patients with Non-Small-Cell Lung Cancer.* Eur Rev Med Pharmacol Sci. 2018;22:1943-47.

94. Deslee, G.; Adair-Kirk, T. L.; Betsuyaku, T.; Woods, J. C.; Moore, C. H.; Gierada, D. S.; Conradi, S. H.; Atkinson, J. J.; Toennies, H. M.; Battaile, J. T.; Kobayashi, D. K.; Patterson, G. A.; Holtzman, M. J.; Pierce, R. A. *Cigarette Smoke Induces Nucleic-Acid Oxidation in Lung Fibroblasts.* Am J Respir Cell Mol Biol. 2010;43:576-84.

95. Dutra-Tavares, A. C.; Silva, J. O.; Nunes-Freitas, A. L.; Guimarães, V. M. S.; Araújo, U. C.; Conceição, E. P. S.; Moura, E. G.; Lisboa, P. C.; Filgueiras, C. C.; Manhães, A. C.; Abreu-Villaça, Y.; Ribeiro-Carvalho, A. *Maternal Undernutrition During Lactation Alters Nicotine Reward and DOPAC/Dopamine Ratio in Cerebral*

Cortex in Adolescent Mice but Does Not Affect Nicotine-Induced nAChRs Upregulation. Int J Dev Neurosci. 2017;65:45-53.

96. Warren, G. W.; Romano, M. A.; Kudrimoti, M. R.; Randall, M. E.; McGarry, R. C.; Singh, A. K.; Rangnekar, V. M. *Nicotinic Modulation of Therapeutic Response in Vitro and in Vivo.* Int J Cancer. 2012;131:2519-27.

97. Biran, A.; Brownstein, M.; Haklai, R.; Kloog, Y. *Downregulation of Survivin and Aurora A by Histone Deacetylase and RAS Inhibitors: A New Drug Combination for Cancer Therapy.* Int J Cancer, 2011;128:691-701.

98. Gelinas, J. C.; Lewis, N. C.; Harper, M. I.; Melzer, B.; Agar, G.; Rolf, J. D.; Eves, N. D. *Aerobic Exercise Training Does not Alter Vascular Structure and Function in Chronic Obstructive Pulmonary Disease.* Exp Physiol. 2017;102:1548-60.

99. Lu, M.; Lu, J.; Yang, X.; Yang, M.; Tan, H.; Yun, B.; Shi, L. *Association between the NBS1 E185Q Polymorphism and Cancer Risk: A Meta-Analysis.* BMC Cancer. 2009;9:124.

100. Pao, W.; Iafrate, A. J.; Su, Z. *Genetically-Informed Lung Cancer Medicine.* J Pathol. 2011;223:230-40.

101. Dinicola, S.; Morini, V.; Coluccia, P.; Proietti, S.; D'Anselmi, F.; Pasqualato, A.; Masiello, M. G.; Palombo, A.; De Toma, G.; Bizzarri, M.; Cucina, A. *Nicotine Increases Survival in Human Colon Cancer Cells Treated with Chemotherapeutic Drugs.* Toxicol In Vitro. 2013;27:2256-63.

102. Huang, D.; Ma, Z.; He, Y.; Xiao, Y.; Luo, H.; Liang, Q.; Zhong, X.; Bai, J.; He, Z. *Long-Term Cigarette Smoke Exposure Inhibits Histone Deacetylase 2 Expression and Enhances the Nuclear*

Factor-κB Activation in Skeletal Muscle of Mice. Oncotarget. 2017;8:56726-36.

103. Li, M.; Zheng, Y.; Yuan, H.; Liu, Y.; Wen, X. *Effects of Dynamic Changes in Histone Acetylation and Deacetylase Activity on Pulmonary Fibrosis.* Int Immunopharmacol. 2017;52:272-80.

104. Wang, Y. Y.; Liu, Y.; Ni, X. Y.; Bai, Z. H.; Chen, Q. Y.; Zhang, Y.; Gao, F. G. *Nicotine Promotes Cell Proliferation and Induces Resistance to Cisplatin by α7 Nicotinic Acetylcholine Receptor-Mediated Activation in Raw264.7 and El4 Cells.* Oncol Rep. 2014;31:1480-88.

105. John, G.; Kohse, K.; Orasche, J.; Reda, A.; Schnelle-Kreis, J.; Zimmermann, R.; Schmid, O.; Eickelberg, O.; Yildirim, A. Ö. *The Composition of Cigarette Smoke Determines Inflammatory Cell Recruitment to the Lung in COPD Mouse Models.* Clin Sci (Lond) 2014;126:207-21.

106. Petrini, J. H. *The Mre11 Complex and ATM: Collaborating to Navigate S Phase.* Curr Opin Cell Biol. 2000;12:293-6.

107. Davis, R.; Rizwani, W.; Banerjee, S.; Kovacs, M.; Haura, E.; Coppola, D.; Chellappan, S. *Nicotine Promotes Tumor Growth and Metastasis in Mouse Models of Lung Cancer.* PLoS One. 2009;4:e7524.

108. Karran, P. *DNA Double-Strand Break Repair in Mammalian Cells.* Curr Opin Genet Dev. 2000;10:144-50.

109. Du, X. Z.; Li, Q. Y.; Du, F. W.; He, Z. G.; Wang, J. *Sodium Valproate Sensitizes Non-Small Lung Cancer A549 Cells to γδ T-Cell-Mediated Killing through Upregulating the Expression of MICA.* J Biochem Mol Toxicol. 2013;27:492-8.

110. Kim, Y. K.; Seo, D. W.; Kang, D. W.; Lee, H. Y.; Han, J. W.; Kim, S. N. *Involvement of HDAC1 and the PI3K/PKC Signaling Pathways in NF-κB Activation by the HDAC Inhibitor Apicidin.* Biochemical and Biophysical Research Communications. 2006;347:1088-93.

111. Jenkins, C. *Drugs for Chronic Obstructive Pulmonary Disease.* Australian Prescriber. 2017;40:15-19.

112. Hu, X. F.; He, X. T.; Zhou, K. X.; Zhang, C.; Zhao, W. J.; Zhang, T.; Li, J. L.; Deng, J. P.; Dong, Y. L. *The Analgesic Effects of Triptolide in the Bone Cancer Pain Rats via Inhibiting the Upregulation of HDACs in Spinal Glial Cells.* J Neuroinflammation. 2017;14:213.

113. Chen, Q.; Deeb, R. S.; Ma, Y.; Staudt, M. R.; Crystal, R. G.; Gross, S. S. *Serum Metabolite Biomarkers Discriminate Healthy Smokers from COPD Smokers.* PLoS One 2015;10:e0143937.

114. Chu, B. F.; Karpenko, M. J.; Liu, Z.; Aimiuwu, J.; Villalona-Calero M, A.; Chan, K. K.; Grever, M. R.; Otterson, G. A. *Phase 1 Study of 5-aza-2'-Deoxycytidine in Combination with Valproic Acid in Non-Small-Cell Lung Cancer.* Cancer Chemother Pharmacol. 2013;71:115-21.

115. Deslee, G.; Woods, J. C.; Moore, C.; Conradi, S. H.; Gierada, D. S.; Atkinson, J. J. Battaile, J. T.; Liu, L.; Patterson, G. A.; Adair-Kirk, T. L.; Holtzman, M. J.; Pierce, R. A. *Oxidative Damage to Nucleic Acids in Severe Emphysema.* Chest. 2009;135: 965-74.

116. Lacasse, Y.; Montori, V. M.; Lanthier, C.; Maltis, F. *The Validity of Diagnosing Chronic Obstructive Pulmonary Disease from a Large Administrative Database.* Canadian Respiratory Journal, 2005;12:251-6.

117. Dimitrova, N.; De Lange, T. *Cell Cycle-Dependent Role of MRN at Dysfunctional Telomeres: ATM Signaling-Dependent Induction of Nonhomologous End Joining (NHEJ) in G1 and Resection-Mediated Inhibition of NHEJ in G2.* Mol Cell Biol. 2009;29:5552-63.

118. Myler, L. R.; Gallardo, I. F.; Soniat, M. M.; Deshpande, R. A.; Gonzalez, X. B.; Kim, Y.; Paull, T. T.; Finkelstein, I. J. *Single-Molecule Imaging Reveals How Mre11-Rad50-Nbs1 Initiates DNA Break Repair.* Mol Cell. 2017;67:891-8.

119. Dai, Y.; Zhang, Z.; Xu, L.; Shang, Y.; Lu, R.; Chen, J. *Genetic Polymorphisms of IL17A, TLR4, and P2RX7 and Associations with the Risk of Chronic Obstructive Pulmonary Disease.* Mutation Research/Genetic Toxicology and Environmental Mutagenesis. 2018;829:1-5.

120. Kobayashi, J.; Antoccia, A.; Tauchi, H.; Matsuura, S.; Komatsu, K. *NBS1 and Its Functional Role in the DNA Damage Response.* DNA Repair (Amst). 2004;3:855-61.

121. Dasgupta, P.; Kinkade, R.; Joshi, B.; Decook, C.; Haura, E.; Chellappan, S. *Nicotine Inhibits Apoptosis Induced by Chemotherapeutic Drugs by Up-Regulating XIAP and Survivin.* Proc Natl Acad Sci USA. 2006;103:6332-7.

122. Mashimo, S.; Chubachi, S.; Tsutsumi, A.; Kameyama, N.; Sasaki, M.; Jinzaki, M.; Nakamura, H.; Asano, K.; Reilly, J. J. Jr.; Betsuyaku, T. *Relationship between Diminution of Small Pulmonary Vessels and Emphysema in Chronic Obstructive Pulmonary Disease.* Clinical Imaging. 2017;46:85-90.

123. MacDonagh, L.; Gray, S. G.; Breen, E.; Cuffe, S.; Finn, S. P.; O'Byrne, K. J.; Barr, M. P. *BBI608 Inhibits Cancer Stemness and Reverses Cisplatin Resistance in NSCLC.* Cancer Lett. 2018;428:117-126.

124. Nakayama, T.; Kaneko, M.; Kodama, M.; Nagata, C. *Cigarette Smoke Induces DNA Single-Strand Breaks in Human Cells.* Nature. 1985;314:462-4.

125. Tian, Y.; Sun, C.; Zhang, L.; Pan, Y. *Clinical Significance of miRNA - 106a in Non-Small Cell Lung Cancer Patients who Received Cisplatin Combined with Gemcitabine Chemotherapy.* Cancer Biol Med. 2018;15:157-64.

126. Lee, J. H.; Mand, M. R.; Deshpande, R. A.; Kinoshita, E.; Yang, S. H.; Wyman, C.; Paull, T. T. *Ataxia Telangiectasia-Mutated (ATM) Kinase Activity Is Regulated by ATP-Driven Conformational Changes in the Mre11/Rad50/Nbs1 (MRN) Complex.* J Biol Chem. 2013;288:12840-51.

127. Ceylan, E.; Kocyigit, A.; Gencer, M.; Aksoy, N.; Selek, S. *Increased DNA Damage in Patients with Chronic Obstructive Pulmonary Disease Who Had Once Smoked or Been Exposed to Biomass.* Respir Med 2006;100:1270-6.

128. Li, Y.; Cho, M. H.; Zhou, X. *What Do Polymorphisms Tell Us about the Mechanisms of COPD?* Clin Sci, 2017;131:2847-63.

129. Gu, C.; Li, Y.; Liu, J.; Ying, X.; Liu, Y.; Yan, J.; Chen, C.; Zhou, H.; Cao, L.; Ma, Y. *LncRNA-Mediated SIRT1/FoxO3a and SIRT1/p53 Signaling Pathways Regulate Type 2 Alveolar Epithelial Cell Senescence in Patients with Chronic Obstructive Pulmonary Disease.* Molecular Medicine Reports 2017;15:3129-3134.

130. D'Amours, D.; Jackson, S. P. *The Mre11 Complex: At the Crossroads of DNA Repair and Checkpoint Signalling.* Nat Rev Mol Cell Biol. 2002;3:317-27.

131. Tsubokawa, M.; Tohyama, Y.; Tohyama, K.; Asahi, M.; Inazu, T.; Nakamura, H.; Saito, H.; Yamamura, H. *Interleukin-3 Activates*

Syk in a Human Myeloblastic Leukemia Cell Line, AML193. Eur J Biochem. 1997;249:792-6.

132. Uziel, T.; Lerenthal, Y.; Moyal, L.; Andegeko, Y.; Mittelman, L.; Shiloh, Y. *Requirement of the MRN Complex for ATM Activation by DNA Damage.* EMBO J. 2003;22:5612-21.

133. Vlahos, R.; Bozinovski, S. *Recent Advances in Pre-clinical Mouse Models of COPD.* Clin Sci (Lond). 2014;126:253-65.

134. Wu, L.; Wang, Y.; Liu, Y.; Yu, S.; Xie, H.; Shi, X.; Qin, S.; Ma, F.; Tan, T. Z.; Thiery, J. P.; Chen, L. *A Central Role for TRPS1 in the Control of Cell Cycle and Cancer Development.* Oncotarget. 2014;5:7677-90.

135. Wang, L.; Ma, L.; Xu, F.; Zhai, W.; Dong, S.; Yin, L.; Liu, J.; Yu, Z. *Role of Long Non-Coding RNA in Drug Resistance in Non-Small Cell Lung Cancer.* Thorac Cancer. 2018;9:761-8.

136. Zhang, C.; Yu, P.; Zhu, L.; Zhao, Q.; Lu, X.; Bo, S. Blockade of α7 Nicotinic Acetylcholine Receptors Inhibit Nicotine-Induced Tumor Growth and Vimentin Expression in Non-Small Cell Lung Cancer through MEK/ERK Signaling Way. Oncol Rep. 2017;38:3309-18.

137. Zheng, M. D.; Wang, N. D.; Li, X. L.; Yan, J.; Tang, J. H.; Zhao, X. H.; Zhang, Z. *Toosendanin Mediates Cisplatin Sensitization through Targeting Annexin A4/ATP7A in Non-Small Cell Lung Cancer Cells.* J Nat Med. 2018;72:724-733.

www.ingramcontent.com/pod-product-compliance
Lightning Source LLC
Chambersburg PA
CBHW030838180526
45163CB00004B/1369